YOGA for
CHRONIC PAIN ...
WTF?

*Take Control,
Combat Pain*

&

***ROCK** Your Life!*

SAMANTHA PARKER

Published by Neoteric Movement Systems, Inc.

The phrase "It's all about perspective" is a trademark of Neoteric Movement Systems, Inc.

Parker, Samantha
Yoga for Chronic Pain ... WTF? Take Control, Combat Pain and Rock Your Life
Paperback ISBN: 978-0-692-12267-9
E-book ISBN: 978-0-692-12268-6

Cover design: Joe Potter
Author photos: Leann Weston Photography
Interior design: Deanne Marie

DEDICATION

I want to dedicate this book to all of the patients and clients that encouraged and swore to me that others in the world wanted to hear my smart-ass fun facts, comments and ideas about yoga. And to those of you who actually read this book, if you don't like it ... they told me to do it.

(You all better be right or I'll find you and make you do more inch worms.)

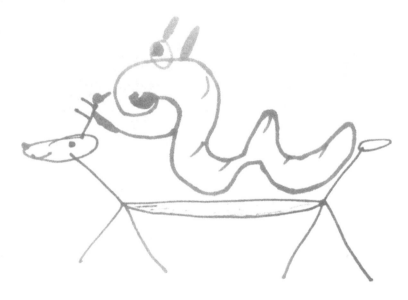

This book is dedicated to all of those who have felt like a misfit in a yoga class. Or thought they would be one if they went to a yoga class.

DISCLAIMER

Everything within this book are my own personal opinions, based on my own research and understanding. The views and opinions expressed herein do not reflect the official policy or views of the United Stated Government, my yoga teachers, or any co-workers past or present.

Always consult your doctor before altering your pain management program, and before starting a yoga practice.

PRAISE FOR YOGA FOR CHRONIC PAIN ... WTF?

Yoga, is some serious sh!t, WTF! Samantha, takes yoga by the horns, wrestles the complex and wins! Her dynamic, in-your-face approach to self-healing is not only refreshing but it's how it MUST be done! Samantha succinctly utilizes her years in *patient care trench warfare* to show you how to get your mental and physical *life back!* As a triple board-certified physician in Anesthesiology, Pain Medicine and Addiction who has seen the failures of opioids and the inadequacy of interventional pain medicine, that I can wholeheartedly say *Yoga for Chronic Pain* is an arrow in my treatment quiver for all my chronic pain patients.

Ronald L. White, MD
U.S. Army, Medical Corp
Lieutenant Colonel (Retired)
Former Chief of Landstuhl Regional Medical Center Interdisciplinary Pain Medicine Department and Founder of the First Pain Intensive Outpatient Program within the Department of Defense

Using these techniques, I'm mentally and physically better. Before Sam's chronic pain program, I had the, "I can't" excuse ready and available. After going through her program, not only have I learned how to physically work through the pain, I've learned how to conquer the mental obstacles.

Will M.
United States Air Force, Retired

In *Yoga for Chronic Pain ... WTF?*, Samantha breaks down the mechanics of chronic pain in a way that I've never seen before. She approaches the issue of chronic pain from a new perspective that anyone can understand, and then uses this new understanding to break free from pain by addressing its source. And she does it in a way that's refreshingly frank and practical. Anyone who has suffered from chronic pain due to any kind of injury can benefit from reading this book and applying its principles, both on the yoga mat and in everyday life.

Larry Broughton
U.S. Army Special Forces
CEO, broughtonHOTELS

As a combat veteran and U.S. Army Special Forces soldier, working with Sam and her program of yoga for chronic pain has helped me tremendously. After being involved in numerous parachute jumps and a hard life of Special Forces training, from walking across mountain peaks with 75+ pounds of equipment in Afghanistan to swimming in frozen lakes in Eastern Europe, my body took a lot of punishment. Sam and her yoga for chronic pain program put me back together. I had two neck surgeries with total disc replacement then total fusion and caging of my neck, as well as a brain surgery. I should not be moving let alone back in the gym. And I owe it all to Sam's yoga for chronic pain. No shit this works. I am a walking testament to this. And I don't put my name on anything that doesn't work. Buy the book, do the program and feel the difference in your life.

Dave T.
U.S. Army Special Forces, Retired

Samantha brings her no-nonsense style that she has in life to the sound advice she provides in this book. After spending over 20 years in the U.S. Army Special Forces, she is exactly who I needed to guide me through my pain and injury management. Those of us who have spent our entire life as "Type-A" personalities normally do not spend a lot of time around yoga studios, which Sam has shown me is an attitude that must change. The benefits I gained from yoga, and in particular Samantha's personal style of yoga, has truly changed the way I look at life and dealing with chronic pain. As a former Green Beret medic and NR-EMT Paramedic, I can attest that Sam's knowledge of healthcare, therapy, and mind and body connectivity is superb.

James C.
U.S. Army Special Forces, Retired

As a 26+ year, decorated combat veteran, who ran multiple marathons and half marathons, I was not able to stand more than 20 minutes due to chronic back pain from an injury in Iraq. I was at the end of my rope when I was introduced to Sam's yoga program for chronic pain. Within weeks of implementing this program, I was fully operational and returned to a status of 100 percent mission ready. This program is saving the Department of Defense millions of dollars by returning highly trained warriors to return to duty. I am so thankful for being introduced to Sam's approach and program.

Major Don "DJ" Jones
United States Air Force, Retired

CONTENTS

ACKNOWLEDGEMENTS

I never would have thought I would have made a career out of yoga. There have been so many that have influenced and have helped me get to this point. That never crossed my mind even after I had been teaching for five years. And now to have written a book??!! So I want to apologize in advance for those that I will forget to mention. I do know that the encouragement from past patients, clients, co-workers, friends, family and strangers who believed in me when I did not believe in myself will never be forgotten. I promise I will keep paying it forward. Karma baby.

First, I want to thank my boys Wylie and Wyatt. They are the best kids ever!! You have taught me more than I feel I have taught you. You are both amazing! Don't ever forget it. (And thank you for thinking my job is cool.) I love you both!!

Jeff Frankart: my mentor, my co-worker, my friend, my ally in encouraging me to step outside the box where I thought belonged. And for actually believing in me that I knew what I was doing. Thank you for all of the words for wisdom, from movement to human nature. You not only have changed my life for the better, but all of the patients and people that have come into your life. You do make a difference in those who want to better their life.

To all of the patients and clients that put up with my squirreling yet plied me with admiration when I finally got to my big idea. Thank you for being real, raw and authentic. You have all taught me so much. Things I could never have learned in a classroom or in a book. Thank you for your encouragement in insisting I needed to open my own yoga dojo and teach people how to teach yoga so you'd have somewhere to go that actually knew what the fuck they were doing. For encouraging me to write this book swearing to me that people would want to listen to me and read it. Let's hope you're right about that. Thank you for bringing and sharing the magic you are into my life. For believing and acknowledging the magical kind of crazy. Please don't forget ... you are the magic.

I want to thank all of my friends who have given me unconditional love, support, and more importantly have supported and encouraged my magical crazy. For giving me that side look out of your eye that I've lost my mind, yet saying, "Go for it."

Larry Broughton for encouraging me with several comments. The first one when I first saw him on stage speaking and during his speech one of the comment was, "If you keep fining yourself saying, 'Hmmm ... what a coincidence.' Stomp Stomp. It's not a coincidence. It's the universe." And, "Wow. You could turkey trot this all kinds of ways." Your friends and your family will encourage you saying you have a great idea. However, when successful professionals are impressed with your idea that is a huge industrial-sized fan that helps to bring the fire embers back to a raging bonfire.

To Syracuse University that provides amazing programs and support for veterans, active duty, women and significant others who support their soldiers while serving their county. And then again as they start to embark into the world of entrepreneurship and starting new chapters in their lives.

To all of those who pointed me in the right direction. To all of those that stood politely listening to me, waiting for me to come up for air, and wondering the whole time, "Does this chick ever stop talking?" For all of those who gave me free advice and even those who charged me for it.

To my fantastic editor, Deanne Marie who is simply amazing in keeping me on track. For your honesty, your kindness, time and guidance. I am sorry that I got you into this. (I can't wait to work with you again!)

To those who advised me to stay on the paved road as I emerged out of the overgrowth, only to cross that paved road to head straight into the overgrowth on the other side, I know your caution came from your own fear but as well as a place of love.

And to all that have underestimated me ... the blonde is bottled.

For those that tried to limit my potential due to their own fears, for doubting me and telling me my ideas were foolish, thank you for pissing me off in making me want to prove you wrong.

Always be open to possibilities.

At no time are we ever broken. We are just under construction.

It's all about perspective.

INTRODUCTION

Good! I got your attention and you are reading this book.

What you don't know is, this is possibly the first step in gaining back control of your chronic pain and your life.

If you have some type of chronic pain at one point in your journey I bet you were advised to start doing yoga. And at one point you said, "WTF?" As in, "My doctor told me to do yoga. WTF?"

Or maybe you've gone to a yoga class on your own because you read online that it would be good for your back. So, you went to a yoga studio, and in participating in the class and you found yourself saying, "WTF? This is my first class. How the hell am I supposed to bend like that?"

Or you have gone to a yoga class, completed the class successfully only to get home and several hours or a day or two later, the underlining reason you went to the class flared up and you're in more pain than when you went to the class! WTF? I thought the class was supposed to help me, not hurt me?

As you read this book, you may find yourself saying, "WTF? Why is she talking about this?" when I get into science and physiology.

The idea is to help you gain better insight and knowledge of how traditional poses can be modified, and to give you a better insight as to what is physically happening to your body when you practice yoga. Yoga can help you gain control of your chronic pain. Having a better understanding of the logic and the rationale of why something works (or doesn't!) and what is going on with you can help prepare you for your yoga practice.

My goal is to take away the mystery, the mystic and the hippie dippy yoga fluff so you will be able to walk away from a yoga session and *implement* what you did on your yoga mat throughout the rest of your day, week and possibly life. They say that half of figuring out what does work, is figuring out what doesn't work.

And if you have been practicing yoga in more traditional ways, and it's not working for you, what have you got too lose by looking at and approaching yoga from a different perspective?

I have been fortunate to have had some amazing job opportunities as a yoga instructor. I have taught thousands of hours of yoga classes, treated thousands of patients, students and clients all who typically have some type of chronic pain. I have worked with professional athletes and many of them have the same concerns and questions as you do when learning and practicing yoga. One thing that I have found to be the most valuable to them, is when the individual understands the logic, the reason and the value why they should do something, they are more inclined to do it. Which will lead to you being more proactive in taking back control of your chronic pain and your life.

Disclaimer! I am NOT a licensed medical provider of any kind. I just use common sense. And a bit of science.

I'm a certified yoga therapist (C-IAYT) with a B.S. in sports and exercise science, and as I write this book, I'm working on my master's degree in kinesiology. I've taught over 6,000 hours of yoga on three different continents, treating thousands of patients.

Much of what you'll read in this book I learned while working as the Chief Movement Therapist at Landstuhl Regional Medical Center—the largest military hospital outside the U.S.—in the Interdisciplinary Pain Management Center. Landstuhl, located in Germany, serves the U.S. military personnel stationed in Europe, and serves as the treatment center for seriously injured soldiers coming out of Iraq and Afghanistan.

As you read this book you may find yourself saying, "WTF? Why is she being such a bitch?" If I come across that way, I apologize. That is not my intent. My intent is to come at this yoga thing from a different angle. Ass backwards. If I were to tell you, "It's okay you poor thing. If you don't want to move, you just stay on the couch. Go into child's pose on your yoga mat. Or just lay there like a slug and don't do anything to help yourself. Inertia will get you healthy."

I would then be labeled as an enabler. And if I am not mistaken there are plenty of people in your life who play that role now, right? *This may be a contributing factor to the physical state that you are in now!* And if so, how's that working for you?

I am not here to make friends. If I do, great. I am not here to tell you everything is going to be okay. I'm here to help and give you guidance. I'm here to arm you with knowledge to help you become functional so you are able to get back to living the life that YOU want. Not the life that your chronic pain is having you lead at the moment.

I'm here to get you back to doing simple mundane sucky tasks around the house like washing dishes and doing the laundry without your back spasming out. So you can go outside and throw a baseball or kick a soccer ball with your kids. So you can get back to a hobby or sport you enjoy. So you can go through a full day of work and when you come home you still have energy to be able to hang out with your family and live life rather than watching it from the couch. So you are able to reach down, pick up your child and hug them. To protect your child from their aspiring dreams of flying and as they leap off the couch pretending to fly like a superhero, so you (out of parental instinct) can leap, dive, roll to their aid and try to buffer their fall before they crack their heads open.

I'm here so you can finally say, ***"Fuck my chronic pain. I will be in charge from here on out!"*** Throughout this book, I'll give you tools that you can use in your yoga practice to start your yoga journey safely, practically, and efficiently. Tools that will help you live the best possible life you can and to take back control of your chronic pain and your life.

Chronic pain can be a beast that can shadow and control your life not only impacting the one with the pain, but of those that you love and are surrounded by, in ways you may not even know.

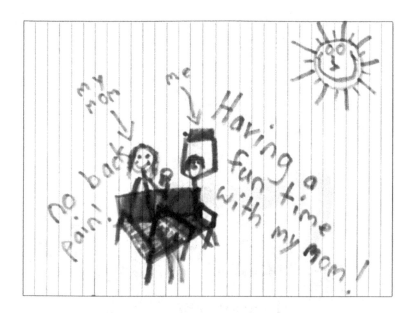

This drawing was done by one of my patient's children. The saying "A picture says a thousand words" is absolutely true! It's why I do what I do.

Remember, *what you put into life is exactly what you are going to get out of it*. I'm not going to lie. It will take effort. It will be challenging. You can keep saying "one day" or make this Day One. The choice is yours.

So, what choice are you going to make?

My sincerest hope for you is that you'll turn the page and start this journey to a pain-free or reduced pain life with me.

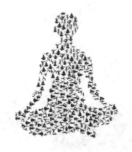

*Yoga is the journey of the self,
through the self,
to the self.*
–The Bhagavad Gita

1

It's All About Perspective ...
Can't is a Choice!

Let me start this book off on the right foot by getting something out of the way: you are no longer allowed to use the word "can't" in your vocabulary. Why? For several reasons. First, it's a negative word that immediately limits our thinking. Second ... I just don't like it. Enough said.

Can't is a *choice*. The minute we tell ourselves that we can't do something, we make it true. Henry Ford once said, "Whether you think you can or think you can't, you're right." Our words have a direct negative or positive effect on not only our minds, but they also trigger major physiological responses, including in our body's immune system (which I will discuss later).

The "C" word is toxic. Eliminate it from your lexicon, because you *can* do it. You'll notice throughout this book I keep mentioning that you have a choice. It's all about perspective.

I live by the belief that if you're having problems accomplishing a goal, you have some choices to make. You either go around it, under it, over it, or as your last resort, you go fucking through it. You may come out bloody on the other side, but those superficial wounds will heal. The lasting, positive changes you choose to make and see through will last you a lifetime.

Why am I telling you this? Because it directly relates to how you practice yoga, how your yoga practice has a direct impact on your chronic pain, and how your yoga practice carries over into your everyday life. In this chapter we'll explore the traditional route than many people take in a yoga practice, and why it just doesn't work for someone trying to relieve chronic pain.

A Day in Your Yoga Life

Tell me if this sounds familiar. You suffer an acute injury of some kind or you find yourself having back, neck, head, or some other kind of pain. It's an "issue" for you. (We are going to call chronic pain and other medical concerns "issues" in this book. We all have issues, but some have more than others.) Maybe a particular incident caused your pain, or maybe you don't even know why you're hurting.

You go to the doctor's office and they tell you that you need to give it some time. Maybe they suggest some possible medical procedures to temporarily block the pain, but they can't guarantee they will work. They suggest some medications that you can take for a short amount of time. Then they recommend doing yoga—"It's great for you!" (Yes, they're right.) But often, that is the only advice you receive about yoga: Just do it.

So you do some research online about this yoga thing, and many of the same poses keep coming up. You get a little confused about the types of yoga out there, so you decide to buy a book. They suggest similar yoga poses, and it appears you can do this on your own at home. You pick a book and place your order.

After you've read the book, you feel like some chapters gave good advice but, overall, following the rules and assuming these poses doesn't seem to have helped your pain that much. Maybe a few poses gave some temporary relief, but your chronic pain is still running your life.

So you decide to find a yoga class. You think going in person and having an instructor teach you may work better for you. You Google and Yelp and come across a local studio that looks nice—the price is right and the classes look like fun, so you sign yourself up.

In anticipation of this new adventure (no—make that "permanent lifestyle change!"), you go shopping to find yourself some cute new yoga clothes. Hell, you even pick up your own yoga mat. You figure you probably don't want to be using rental yoga mats, with someone else's "chi" on it.

Equipped and dressed to impress, you head out to your carefully selected boutique yoga studio. You walk in, soft music plays, maybe there's a hint of essential oils is in the air, and the people there look very fit (not to mention adorable) in their yoga outfits. You think, "Wow, this yoga thing must really work!" And, "Thank goodness I invested in this new yoga outfit and yoga mat so I blend in."

"How long am I going to have to sit here?"
you wail inside.

You take off your shoes and leave them in the cubby by the door, thinking you probably should have made time for that pedicure last weekend. Inside the yoga room, you find a place on the floor, rolling out your very expensive, very stylish yoga mat and sit on it in your equally expensive, equally stylish new two-piece matching yoga outfit. You feel ready to go, even excited.

You think, "Finally, this is going to help my chronic pain! (And I look cute, too.)"

The instructor begins the class, telling everyone to sit still, listen to their bodies, center themselves, let go of expectations, get grounded, and focus on breathing. Sitting there, fighting the urge to move because your back is starting to "speak" very loudly at you, you wonder what all that really means.

"How long am I going to have to sit here?" you wail inside.

You feel the need to shift your weight differently, but you don't dare move, because you're afraid you'll make noise and get yelled at by the instructor for interrupting other people's zen.

You open one eye, trying not to make it obvious that you're looking around the room, to make sure everyone is still sitting and breathing and that you didn't miss something.

"Damn it, how they hell are they able to look so comfortable, sitting with their legs like that?" you wonder.

The instructor finally instructs you to move, and you're flushed with relief. Leading you into pose after pose, she urges you to "take it to your edge" while you "listen to your body." In your mind, you're hearing, "Listen to my body? My body is telling me to get the fuck out of this class and call it a day!"

You have no idea what the fucking "edge" is she's talking about, because if you could see it, you'd more than likely jump off it right now. Your body is screaming at you to stop, grab your mat, and flip everyone the bird on your way out the door.

How the hell are they making it look so easy?

But you tell yourself you're here to give it your best. And you've got to stay, if for no other reason than to make dropping all that money on your new yoga outfit and mat worthwhile. You notice there are several poses, even seemingly easy ones, that right away begin to aggravate your problem areas. It doesn't feel quite right, and at times it just *hurts*.

You go to your knees, looking around to see what everyone else is doing. How the hell are they making it look so easy? You realize that you are in way over your head.

You look around, thinking, "They've lost their ever-loving-minds if they think I'm going to be contorting my body into that pose anytime soon." But once again, the guilt you feel for spending entirely too much money on yoga gear creeps in, and you attempt most of the poses anyway, because your conscience is telling you that you need to.

You finish the class, feeling a little overwhelmed but proud of yourself for sticking it out. You didn't give in, and you didn't run. But you're also thinking that this type of torture must have been invented by some kind of sadist. You've already decided that you're never doing yoga again. Screw that!

You go home and open a bottle of wine, meanwhile devising your own version of a sun salutation ... with your wine glass to your lips. And then that harder-than-it-looks *savasana* ... in your bed! The next morning, you roll out of bed the feeling twinges of pain/hurt/discomfort and, as the day goes on, that feeling worsens. You went to yoga to help fix your issue, but now it's even worse. That's it—no more!

Guess what? You're not alone. This happens every day between well-intentioned yoga instructors and eager-to-learn students. Yoga really can help so many. However, while a lot of instructors are out there trying to help, they unfortunately do not have the knowledge or experience to cue and instruct those who are suffering from certain medical issues.

There are ways to modify poses in the beginning that will help you work your way up to what I like to call "optimal yoga pose potential," or OYPP. The yoga community is deceiving you if you're learning that the more you practice yoga, the closer you'll get to OYPP. The truth is, many will never reach OYPP because of genetics, biomechanics, or injuries that they have sustained throughout their lives. And guess what? You don't *need* to reach OYPP. I personally think that many of those poses are just plain creepy. I don't see how or why they are good for the body, with my understanding of anatomy and physiology.

Making OYPP the goal is not helpful. Trying to achieve it could potentially cause you harm. And the main question really becomes, *why* are you trying to achieve OYPP? Many times, it's just a pesky ego telling you that if you want to "fit in," you need to reach OYPP. Bullshit. In fact, that kind of thinking is the opposite of what yoga is all about.

Doing No Harm

Yoga is believed to have been around for the past 3,000 to 4,000 years depending on who you talk to. Originating in India, yoga is a practice of bringing harmony, balance and spirituality between the mind and body. The word *yoga* comes from the Sanskrit word *yuj* meaning to join, yoke or unite.

Thus, a yoga practitioner sets out on this journey to unite their individual consciousness with the Universal Consciousness in hopes of reaching self-realization bringing harmony between mind and body, between man and nature.

For those fairly new to yoga, here's a crash course in some underlying principles and guidelines from the yoga perspective.

There are five *yamas*—ethical, moral and societal guidelines for living a meaningful, purposeful life. If you're a Christian, you'll find yamas very similar to the Ten Commandments. But keep in mind, yoga is not a religion! It's a way for some people to gain spirituality in their lives ... very similar to religion, but still two *completely* different things.

One of these yamas, considered the most important by most yogis, is *ahimsa,* which is the Sanskrit word for nonviolence or "non-injury." Other yamas include *satya,* or truthfulness; *asteya,* non-stealing; *brahmacharya,* continence; and *apaigraha,* non-covetousness. (Sound familiar to your religious beliefs? It's very much like the Golden Rule: "Do unto others ....")

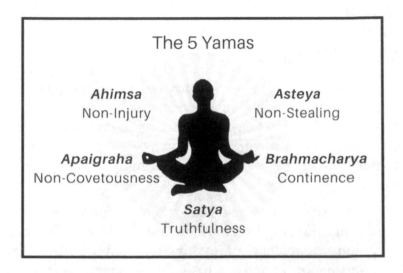

Ahimsa, which can be loosely translated to "Do no harm," is the primary underlying philosophy of yoga. The documentary *Yoga Unveiled* tells the stories of many of the founding fathers of yoga. Watching that documentary, I was struck by this vow to do no harm.

Think about this: Yoga has been around for 4,000 years give or take. The local yogis were the original medicine men, the village doctors. Ahimsa was essentially their Hippocratic

Oath. Yoga is about healing, not hurting—physically, mentally, and emotionally—causing no harm to yourself or to others.

We can relate ahimsa to thoughts and actions not only toward others but also ourselves. Maybe on that first day of yoga class, you allowed your ego to creep in and take over (gasp!). And maybe that's why you rolled out of bed the next day so sore or with your chronic pain flaring up.

If we truly practice ahimsa, nonviolence also means not causing harm to ourselves.

Often, as we try to be "good little students," we push ourselves to do exactly what the instructor is telling us to do, even as our bodies are telling us things like,

"Don't go so far."

"Ease off!"

"I'm really not ready for that."

We feel compelled to try to do the moves perfectly, and sometimes we actually hurt ourselves. Why do we do that? If we truly practice ahimsa, nonviolence also means not causing harm to ourselves. When we let our egos convince us that we have to push ourselves unreasonably to get in a good workout, we're not adhering to the principle of ahimsa.

You might be tempted to blame your pushing yourself on the yoga instructor, because he or she says things like, "Take yourself to your edge!" or "Reach back as far as you can, go deep, and breathe."

Most instructors out there really do want to give their clients the opportunity to get a good workout. In fact, you can find "power yoga," "blast-off yoga," and other similarly titled classes that target those who are looking for a hard workout with maximum benefits. In these classes, instructors typically take you through the movements quickly, work you up to a "peak pose" (one that is very challenging), and might even instruct you to go into a headstand. A few things you should know about these "power" classes:

• You will sweat more in these classes, because you're trying to keep up, rushing to get into the next pose.

• The momentum of moving so fast actually helps you "cheat," and you aren't working your muscles as intensely as you would be if you moved slower.

• The hazard of moving fast and worrying about getting into the next pose is that you're not being as present and as mindful as you should be.

If you suffer from chronic pain, it is *extremely* important for you to be aware of what your body it telling you. Mainly because if you have chronic pain, then your central nervous system is somewhat "out of whack" and is likely giving you improper feedback. So it is even more important to slow things down and pay attention to your form and how your body is feeling. I'll go deeper into this topic in upcoming chapters.

The disclaimer of "listen to your body" is not enough for people with chronic pain.

Many instructors teaching these power classes lack a good understanding of anatomy and physiology (not all, but many). Some believe that asking the entire class to do a headstand if it is part of the student's practice (but telling them to listen to their bodies and don't do it if they don't want to) is proper teaching. For advanced students, it is.

But the disclaimer of "listen to your body" is not enough for beginning students and especially for people with chronic pain. And far too many students believe they are "advanced" when they are not!

The majority of people seeking yoga are in need of yoga's healing power. Now, I won't be surprised if I receive angry e-mails and letters about this, but the yoga instructors who push power yoga are tailoring their classes to the student's perception that they are intermediate or advanced. They are teaching to the minorities of the world, not the majority of people who walk into their classes.

You are the normal (if there can be a "normal"), average person going to a yoga class. The cute, shapely people that can do the handstands, who have worked very hard to get where they are, and whose dedication is certainly commendable—they are the minority.

People who regularly practice yoga start for various reasons, but most are looking to see and feel the physical benefit. For some, it's simply to be able to once again fit into their favorite jeans. But for many, just like you, it's a serious effort to combat their chronic pain so they can feel better, work better and live better.

I've learned to ask myself,
"Is what I am doing going to cause me harm?"

Pushing ourselves beyond what is sensible is something everyone has to keep in check— instructors and students alike. We all fall prey to our egos telling us that we can (and we must!) do what is being asked of us, even if our bodies are clearly telling us not to push so hard that day. But when we give in to our egos, we are ignoring the tenet of "do no harm"—we're rejecting ahimsa as it relates to our own bodies.

Please, do not confuse doing no harm with the limiting thought that you can't do something! As I said at the beginning of this chapter, it's all about perspective.

We can do the poses that the other yoga Barbies are doing in the class. We just won't look like them. We may eventually get our bodies to contort and perform like theirs, but it may also never happen for some. We are all genetically different thank goodness! (I don't know about you, but I don't think the world could handle a couple of me walking around!) Even if genetics is factored out, and you have sustained an injury that others have not, you may never be able to achieve OYPP. And guess what? *That's fine.* You will still be able to benefit from your modified yoga poses. You will still be able to control and manage your chronic pain with yoga if you choose to do so.

I admit, I'm a recovering OFA (over-fucking achiever) and it is extremely hard to check my ego at the door, listen to my body, and ease up when I should. It's a constant struggle for me. So, while practicing, I've learned to ask myself, "Is what

I am doing going to cause me harm?" I find myself often providing verbal cues, "It's okay to ease off and go to child's pose." Or, "There is no gain pushing through the pain."

I want to live a long, healthy and active life. I know that if I push myself to my own personal "edge" too many times, it will inevitably result in injury at some point. Don't get me wrong: I *do* believe that you need to incorporate a vigorous yoga practice into your regular routine. A powerful workout can provide excellent benefits and is necessary for strengthening and training your body. Yoga is a tool to help us heal on many different levels. It's both proactive and reactive medicine for the mind, body, heart, and soul.

It's been a hard lesson for me to learn, to teach, and to uphold, that it is okay to back off if you feel like you should. I frequently hear my students regretfully admitting, "I knew I should have eased off, but I didn't. It's my own fault." I like to hear them take responsibility for and ownership of their actions. Stopping before we push ourselves too far is one of the hardest, yet most important, things we can do as we practice yoga. But once we understand the importance of taking care to protect our bodies, it puts us in the driver's seat, in complete control of steering our "vehicles" in the direction we want to go.

Taking Ownership of Our Choices

In yoga and in life, every choice has a consequence, either positive or negative. I taught my children that from a very early age. For example, in the following scenario, they have a choice to make and there are consequences:

1. Clean your room now, and then you can watch television; or

2. Clean your room when you want to, and you will not get to watch television today.

Each of these choices results in either a positive or a negative consequence.

Ownership of our actions gives us power!

The same holds true for grown-ups. We must own the fact that we are the only ones in control of our actions and reactions to the world around us and, if we make a choice, the consequences are on us. If we choose to push ourselves to our edge—or not to practice at all—and we pay the price with physical pain, we have only ourselves to blame.

However, I choose to look at this from this perspective: **ownership of our actions gives us power!** We can turn our weaknesses into strengths when we identify what we have to work on, then make a conscious effort to correct those thoughts, actions, or behaviors.

Taking an honest look at your behavior and decisions, both on and off the mat, may even identify factors within your control that are contributing to your chronic pain.

Your instructor is up there leading you, but you are always responsible for your own body. Your instructor can't feel your pain and doesn't know your exact limits, so he or she is not the best person to make decisions about how much you should or shouldn't do.

The most important thing you need to do in the studio is tune into your body to learn how to best manage your chronic pain and keep yourself safe. That's exactly what I'm going to show you in this book. But first, let's dive into what chronic pain is, and why there are no quick fixes.

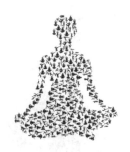

*Nothing ever goes away
until it has taught us
what we need to know.*
–Pema Chodron

2

The Real Cost of Chronic Pain

There may be times when you feel like you are alone with your chronic pain. You may feel a bit isolated when you are invited to hang out with friends. Or when your family wants you to go on a hike with them, or to the park, or to take a bike ride.

Because as much as you would like to participate in these activities, when your back pain flares up, or you are on the verge of a migraine, you know you're risking making those conditions worse if you push yourself.

On the other hand, taking care of yourself and knowing your limits can leave you frustrated and alone, sometimes even depressed.

The struggle is real. I get it.

The same thing can happen at work. You're doing your best to make it through the day and to get your work done on time. You push through your pain and discomfort to create a fantastic presentation and you're relieved. You made it! Your co-workers ask you to join them for a celebratory drink to toast the team landing that new client. You want to be a team player, but you know if you sit on that barstool too long, by the time you get home you'll be pushing through your pain even more as you try to give your young child a bath.

Hell, you barely got that presentation done in time, and you're exhausted and your body is screaming at you to give it some TLC!

You feel that you're not able to live your life the way you want to, because this pain/discomfort limits your actions and forces you to make choices that you would rather not be making. It limits your fun. It limits your adventure and it just pisses you off!

You, my friend, are not alone. Not by a long shot.

This chapter might just blow your mind when you realize how big of a problem chronic pain really is—and what might actually be causing it.

What Chronic Pain Is ... and Isn't

According to the American Academy of Pain Medicine, 100 million Americans—40 percent of adults—suffer with chronic pain. That's is more than diabetes, heart disease and cancer combined!

Chronic pain can stem from a wide variety of medical issues: injuries, diabetes, other diseases, and just plain old deconditioning and being overweight. Chronic pain can be the result of constantly making poor choices of how we move (or not) throughout our day, what we eat, how much water we drink and how much sleep we get.

Chronic pain can also be difficult to classify, diagnose and treat.

Basically, chronic pain can stem from how we treat our bodies.

Let's define chronic pain. Generally speaking, chronic pain is a pain that last and persists longer than three to six months.[1] The pain becomes progressively worse and occurs on a fairly frequent basis usually outlasting the typical amount of time for injured tissue to heal.

Chronic pain can also be difficult to classify, diagnose and treat. Chronic pain if often described as a hyperactive central nervous system ("CNS" – I'll use this abbreviation a lot) that can affect one in three patients.

An *acute pain* is different from chronic pain. An acute pain is typically brought on by a specific injury, disease or some other type of physical and biological incident. Acute pain is a normal, natural and necessary sensation. This pain is needed to send signals to the brain telling it that something is not right and we need to stop what we're doing. If we don't, we could cause permanent harm and damage. If this acute pain was brought on by an accident that was beyond our control, then it's the alarm bell to the brain saying that you require immediate attention.

Unfortunately, many times there is really no clear cause as to what creates chronic pain and how to deal with it. The medical community is noticing a correlation between how long a patient waits to get moving after an injury and the chance of them developing chronic pain increases, *and* that movement is hugely successful in combating chronic pain. Along with movement, re-evaluating your pain is needed to be successful in combating chronic pain.

Chronic pain has a bunch of other effects, too. Medical professionals have seen that along with chronic pain comes depression, sleep disturbance, mood changes, multiple other health problems, kinesiophobia, hypersensitivity and an overactive central nervous system.

They also realize that many times the only way to try to treat this chronic pain is to throw pain medications at it. (Which, by the way, leads to accidental opioid addictions and deaths. You many have heard we have an opioid epidemic?)

Medical providers are aware that they really should prescribe limited amounts of opioid pain medications, and that there are only so many refills they can give you before you will start to build up a tolerance to it. When a patient is telling them that they are still in pain, the doctors do believe it. But they also understand that more than likely it's not the actual injury that is causing the pain. Its how the patient's brain is now *perceiving* the pain. (I explain this in Chapter 4.) However, if they do not continue to prescribe these pain medications, many patients will start to go doctor shopping—a sure sign of opioid addiction. The truth is, they really have nothing to give you to help diminish the pain while at the same time weaning you of the medication except in extreme circumstances.

When they finally recommend doing yoga, massage therapy, or acupuncture, the patient looks at them like the doctor didn't hear a damn thing they just said.

"I'm in pain. How am I supposed to move?! I need my pills!"

In Chapter 4 I'll explain why you think you are in pain, when in reality your CNS is in overdrive.

Here's the thing: pain medication is BIG business. Think for a moment. How many commercials are you constantly bombarded with for the newest and best pill that will "fix" your problem? (Never mind the two minutes of very fast low-talking with a shit-ton of potential problems that may arise if you decide that this drug is for you.) I bet you see a lot of these ads. And it makes total sense. Pharmaceutical companies are making a fucking fortune!

After just saying that, I do believe there is a need and a time for these drugs. However, I personally think that many who take these drugs need them for much shorter periods of time than they are being prescribed for. And I personally think that way too many people want to take the easy way out with a pill instead of actually going to the gym and eating a carrot.

There is no quick fix!

America has been buying into this idea that life shouldn't be hard. You deserve everything that you want and should have it. After all, this is America. Land of the free, home of the brave and entitled. Marketing companies and pharmaceutical companies know this. So they are selling to that warped consumer mindset.

Pharmaceutical companies and the other companies that want to sell you their products and market them that you be losing weight and inches, you'll be pain free in no time, and you'll fall in love and the world will be filled with rainbows and ponies (beer, wine and beaches full of babes in bikinis for those who have those dreams).

I can't really blame these pharmaceutical companies for filling your heads with the possibility of a quick fix, because many Americans are lazy and don't want to work hard for anything. Americans think that they are entitled to be pain free. Or entitled to have free school. Or entitled to free food. Why do you feel entitled to anything that you did not work for?

Is this sounding like a bit much? Good! No one owes you anything. And the only person that will get you what you want is you. It's the same concept with your pain. The only person truly responsible for your pain is *you*.

There is no quick fix. There is no magic pill.
The magic is YOU.

I hate to be the bearer of bad news, but the pharmaceutical companies are lying to you. Plain and simple. They're full of shit and they want to sell you their product because they want to make money. I don't blame them. Everyone wants to make money. It's reality. Now before you start telling me that you took some pill or tried this weight loss program and it worked, ask yourself if you were able to sustain it? Were you able to implement long lasting sustainable habits to keep the weight off, or to make your pain disappear? Here's another reality: there is no quick fix! There is no magic pill, or diet or workout program.

The magic is when you decide to make the hard right decisions in moving your body, eating better, getting more sleep, drinking more water and decompressing on a more regular basis.

The magic is YOU.

Time to Own Up

Why am I speaking about this and what does it have to do with your chronic pain and yoga?

You are the one buying the product. You are the one looking for the quick fix and want someone else to do the hard work. NO? Okay. Let me ask you a few questions:

When was the last time you went to the gym or got any type of physical activity that did not involve you getting from point A to point B without having to include an errand or getting your kids to soccer practice or to work?

When was the last time you got at least four 30-minute exercise sessions in a week?

When was the last time you ate two pieces of fruit and four serving of vegetables in a day? (And no, French fries don't count as a vegetable.)

How much water did you drink today? Half your body weight in ounces a day? On top of and in addition to any caffeine or alcohol? You were on point today. Great! How was yesterday? Or the day before? (FYI, dehydration can lead to headaches and migraines, dry vertebral discs, and dry scar tissue.)

When was the last time you had soda?

When was the last time you got seven to nine hours of uninterrupted sleep?

These are all factors and actions in your daily life that play a direct role with your chronic pain. Many people say they understand the importance of these factors, but really do not implement them. They say they know they need to do these things for an overall total body wellbeing. Yet, we only do one or two things a week, expect it to work and if it doesn't, oh well, it's not me, I tried. I'll take the pill instead.

Why do you keep choosing to NOT take action?

When you finally own up to the fact that you are in control of your chronic pain and that there are things that you can do—things that are within your power to help alleviate some of this pain—then you are able to free yourself from jumping on the bandwagon of the newest and best workout program or fad diet.

Once again so I'm clear, I am NOT saying that there is no need for pharmaceuticals and medications. There are some people with medical conditions that will have to take meds for the rest of their lives. That's fine. But if you have the power to make choices that may help you come off some of these drugs, lower your health care costs, and be able to spend more time with your family, why do you keep choosing to NOT take action? (Oh, shit just got deep. I'll get a little more into the underlying psychology of this in Chapter 8.)

The Elephant in the Chronic Pain Room

You may or may not be aware that there is an obesity epidemic which affects one in three adults in America. These individuals who are obese have a Body Mass Index (BMI) of 30 and over. Sugary, processed, instant food and beverages are literally at our finger tips whenever and wherever we want. And even though we all know this about the food we eat, we still keep making the same choice of eating crap that isn't good for us.

I personally believe in self-acceptance, loving and accepting ourselves for who we are. However, society is constantly in our faces that you need to have a bigger butt, or bigger lips, bigger meals, or that it is okay to be morbidly obese—just embrace yourself!

As much as I would like to get on this bandwagon, I do not agree with it. I don't believe in body shaming at all, I'm just concerned about our overall health. When I look at a morbidly obese or overweight individual I see their internal organs. I see them walking with an altered gait and I notice the angle of their knees, hips and ankles that are having to handle a load at an angle that the joint is not designed to carry. I see them rubbing their lower back trying to alleviate their pain or see them breathing heavily just walking up a flight of stairs. I would even bet money that these same individuals do not sleep well at night.

When I see these individuals, they do not look like an individual having the fun great life that society and marketing companies are trying to sell us. I'm not buying. I see someone who is struggling on a daily basis, lying to themselves that their lives are great so they feel better about themselves as they keep making shitty choices because it is easier and makes them feel good in the moment.

I feel sorry for these people. I see the life that they are missing out on. I look at them and I see the potential of who they can become.

I am bringing up the obesity epidemic because being obese directly relates too many people's chronic pain. Obesity is the second cause to premature death after smoking. (In Chapter 9 I'll go into more of how being obese relates to your chronic pain and your yoga practice.)

Hopefully now you have a better understanding of what chronic pain is and how much it not only costs the government and businesses, but the cost to you, and I don't just mean the money you lose when you run out of sick days. Even more important than money, it costs you quality time with your loved ones. Something you are not able to put a price on.

The tricky thing about chronic pain is that everyone has a different pain threshold. It can depend on the person's genetics, their physical activity level before chronic pain set in or the injury happened. It can depend on their environment, their physical activity when they were younger, psychological mindset, motivation, cultural and social backgrounds and current situations.

Everyone has a different pain scale and where their zero is. Why? Because everyone is different. In the next chapter I'll explain how to set your personal pain scale.

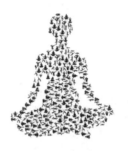

Pain is inevitable.
Suffering is optional.
–Haruki Murakami

3

Resetting Your Pain Scale

One of the first things that you need to do to get a handle on your chronic pain is to reset your pain scale. What is a pain scale? I'm so glad you asked. More than likely, you have been exposed to it at the doctor's office.

You see your primary physician or a nurse for your pain and they ask you, "What face represents your pain today?" There is a row of sad faces, crying faces and happy faces. That pain scale basically grades your pain from zero to ten—zero being no pain to ten being the worst pain you've ever had.

Does this look familiar?

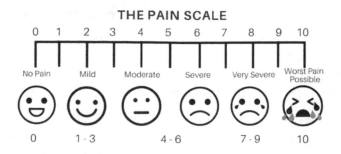

The reason they are asking you this is to gauge just exactly how you perceive your discomfort/pain. At the same time, they are watching how you carry yourself, if you're showing outward signs of physical discomfort, or if you're possibly overcompensating. They may be trying to figure out if what you think is pain is just gas. (Not that gas can't be painful—it can!)

But you all agree this is definitely not gas. You give a rating of somewhere between 7 and 9. Meanwhile, you're thinking to yourself, "All I know is, I'm in a shit-ton of pain. That's why I'm here!" But the more specific and more important question you should be asking yourself is, when you think about yesterday morning and all the mornings last week, which smiley face represents the level of pain you typically wake up with? Maybe somewhere between 3 and 6?

Is your pain level today possibly elevated because of your activity yesterday? Is this simply a flare up today that may subside in a day or two?

"But," you say, "I'm in pain every day." I believe you. Your doctors believe you, too.

Typically, people with chronic pain wake up on a daily basis with pain that is between 2 and 6 on the pain scale, depending on the person and their pain threshold. Everyone is different, of course, and based on their experiences and physical conditioning, both before and after their injury, one person's pain tolerance may be higher than another's.

But if you wake up every day with pain in the range of 3 to 7, then consider *that* number (or that range) your new zero. What I mean by this is, if this pain between 2 and 6 is pretty much an everyday occurrence, then this is what you should consider your "normal" pain level, your starting point, *your* zero.

Now, I know you may be saying to yourself, "Wait, I have pain. How can this be my 'no pain' level?"

What is happening is that, because you have chronic pain, your perception of that pain is being misinterpreted by your brain. In the next chapter I'll be talking about neuroplasticity and what I mean by your brain interpreting your pain to be much greater than it actually is.

Think of your pain like the dimmer switch on a light fixture. If you have little or no pain, that dimmer switch is turned off. You're in sexy mood lighting mode. Once you start to turn the dial up, your pain increases. If you turn the knob all the way up, you are in need of the ER.

So, when your CNS is in overdrive, the wiring in your dimmer switch is telling your brain that the light is in ER mode when it's actually not.

Is It Pain or Discomfort?

Here is a scenario. It's the first of the year and you resolve you're going to drop that last ten pounds. This is the year you're going to do it. You can feel it! You go to the gym fighting to get on the machines and you're doing pretty well for the first couple of days. But you wake up in the morning and you feel muscles you never thought existed let alone could be that sore.

Later in the day when you go to the bathroom you need to go into a handicap stall so you can use the handrail to help you sit down on the toilet after a leg day. Or the yoga class that was all about arm balances. The day after you're lucky to get your arms up high enough to wash your hair. That is perceived by some as pain. Well, it's not. You're just uncomfortable.

And now you are saying, "No! That IS pain."

No, you are just uncomfortable. Maybe extremely uncomfortable, but just uncomfortable.

I get it. We are all human and we do not like to be uncomfortable. Mentally, physically or emotionally. But there is NO growth without discomfort and failure. So you need to ask yourself the question, is the discomfort that will come with being fat, overweight, possibly getting diabetes going to be more painful? Is lower back pain (that will inevitably come when you do not exercise to strengthen your muscles) worth NOT being comfortable for a little while? Is the quality of life that you would be leading the quality of life that you want if you have to watch it from the couch? I'm going off a hunch and saying no.

Look at this discomfort as a positive.

What most people do not understand is that discomfort will go away after a while. You are experiencing a hypersensitivity and DOMS, otherwise known as Delayed Onset Muscle Soreness, and this perfectly normal. In fact, congratulations—you got a good workout! This is going to happen and will continue to happen as you keep increasing your physical activity. And this is a good thing! It means you're not wasting your time while you are in the gym.

The other good thing about this discomfort is that it is temporary! This feeling of "pain" will go away in the next 24 to 72 hours. And as you continue to exercise the hypersensitivity will decrease as well. Look at this discomfort as a positive. You are just building a healthier, stronger body AND desensitizing yourself.

Put Your Pain into Perspective

Back to the pain scale. Thinking back to the day after that Boot Camp class where you ran bleachers or the Power Yoga class where you were doing lots of *chatagungas*, side planks, crows, and your arms were barely allowing you to wash your hair the next day. Where would you put yourself on the pain scale? And do you wake up with this pain on a daily basis?

*You need to look at this pain from
a different perspective.*

There will be some reading this book and say, "I have TRUE REAL pain. Not the kind of muscle soreness that happens after leg day!!" First off, good. I'm glad you can tell the difference. That is many times the first place that you need to be honest with yourself. So thinking back to the muscle soreness, where do you put yourself on that pain scale every day when you wake up? A 5? If so, you pop Motrin, put on a little Icy Hot and off you go.

Now what if you woke up every day and your pain is at 5, due to a lower back issue. Or a neck issue due to a car accident. Or a slip and fall on the ice. Then the same concept comes into play that the 5 pain you feel becomes your new zero. Now, based off of that *new zero*, how is your pain?

I know you may be thinking right now that this doesn't help you gain back control of your chronic pain. But it does. You need to look at this pain from a different perspective.

There are a lot of people who have been dealt some crappy hands. I have worked with many of them. I had an amazing job where I was able to work with military members and many Special Ops as well. Most putting their lives on the line defending our country and our freedoms so that we are safe and are able to have the freedoms we do. (For example, choosing the crappy food that we put into our bodies on a regular basis and not exercising.)

Some of these individuals have been blown up and are missing limbs. Some have been shot numerous times. One of these individuals had his spine reconstructed with a metal cage that was then drilled into his ribs to secure it. (See photo on the following page.) The injury took place when a fellow team mate lost control during a HALO (high altitude, low opening) jump and crashed into him right between the shoulder blades.

There was another individual who had two neck surgeries with total disc replacements, and then a total fusion and the caging put into his neck. Oh, and brain surgery, too. At first all he really wanted to do it to get back to being physically,

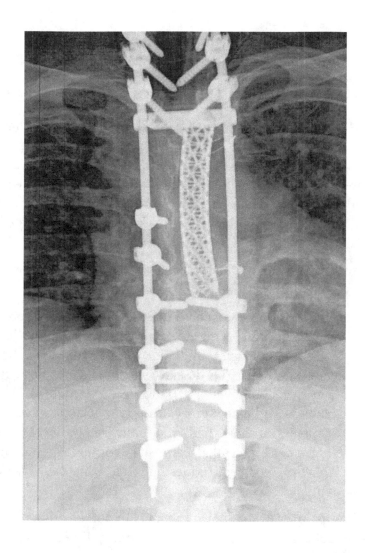

And you say that your lower back is sore because you sit at a desk all day and then choose not to exercise?

mentally and emotionally well again so he could work with his team doing what he loved and trained so hard to do. Keep our county safe. Keep YOU safe. Now all he wants is for the constant headaches to subside even for just a day.

These are just few of the many amazing soldiers that I have had the privilege of working with. These individuals experience pain. And they will every day of their lives. However, resetting their pain scales, and implementing what I address in this book, help them to diminish their pain so they are able to sit with their families at the end of the day and eat dinner. Or to go canoeing with their dog.

And you say that your lower back is sore because you sit at a desk all day and then choose not to exercise?

See, it's all about perspective. Everyone has a different pain scale. I'm not trying to diminish your pain. Your experiences are different than theirs. But ask yourself ... how bad is your pain really? Or do excuses, your fear of flare ups or more pain with movement (kinesiophobia) which leads you to laziness and a sedentary lifestyle tend to lead you to the conclusion of how bad you pain really is? In the psychology world it's called pain catastrophizing. And this catastrophizing feeds your kinesiophobia, which is a fear of movement.

This pain cycle of kinesiophobia, hypersensitivity, and catastrophizing, and then avoidance many times starts off with an over stimulated central nervous system whose dimmer switch is stuck on the high beams.

(Don't think I don't know where some of your minds just went with that last statement. But if it keeps you reading then keep thinking of those high beams shining.)

That's exactly where we're going next—on a little tour of your central nervous system. But first, I really encourage you get a good night's sleep and then notice how your body feels when you wake up. Take out the pain scale at the beginning of this chapter and set your new zero on your personal pain scale.

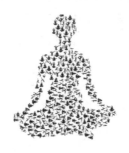

*Insanity is doing
the same thing
over and over again
and expecting
different results.*
– Attributed to Albert Einstein

4

Neuroplasticity and Rebooting Your Brain

You might be thinking to yourself, "What the heck is neuroplasticity and why is this lady talking about something so medical?" Let me explain. Neuroplasticity is a medical buzz word of the day and plays a huge role in our perception of pain.

If you'll bear with me for a bit of a biology lesson (this is about as science-y as I get), I want to help you understand what's going on in your brain when you experience pain sensations. Once you get that, improving your pain by changing your brain will make a lot more sense.

Essentially, we have created these patterns—our habits—throughout our everyday life, sometimes with effort and sometimes without even realizing that we were creating patterns and habits. You may have a fear of clowns based off of an experience you had at friend's birthday party, or even as an adult at a Halloween party. (I never had a bad experience, I just think clowns are creepy.)

45

For example, let's say you're right-handed and you sprain your right wrist. While your wrist is healing, at first you might reach for something with your right hand, only to realize you can't use it. You pause for a moment, then switch to your left hand to reach for the item. It feels awkward at first, but after a week or so, it no longer feels strange. That's neuroplasticity. Your brain learned from its experiences.

The healthier your brain and body are the faster the neurons (nerve cells) in the brain can adapt when injury or disease happen.

Neuroplasticity is what has helped humans over time adapt to the ever-changing environmental, physiological changes and pressures. In the cave man days, living was mostly about survival and keeping the human species alive. If something was trying to get you and kill you, you would learn from previous mistakes of how you were almost some animal's dinner, change your behavior or your patterns so you don't get so close to getting killed on the next hunt. This is learning from your experiences. That's neuroplasticity in action.

Neuroplasticity is what allows the brain to adapt to changes that are inflicted on it by damage and stress. Neuroplasticity also allows us to adapt to just about any and all experiences that we encounter in our lives. It helps us to respond differently and reflexively to situations and circumstances that have been genetically hard wired into us.

Brain Chemistry 101

I'm going to throw a couple of definitions at you that we'll use throughout this chapter.

The Oxford dictionary defines neuroplasticity as "the ability of the brain to form and reorganize synaptic connections, especially in response to learning or experience or following injury."

Neuroplasticity allows the neurons (nerve cells) in the brain to compensate for injury and disease and to adjust their activities in response to new situations or to changes in their environment.

Neurons, which are basic functional units of the brain, relay information throughout the body by electrical signals. In the brain single neurons are required for even the simplest tasks yet they really have no power when they are by themselves. Even these simple tasks require a huge number of interconnected neurons to function as a whole.

How the brain completes each task or responds to a particular situation has been imprinted like ruts in a dirt road into our brains by a unique pattern of connections that fire in a specific sequence for us to respond appropriately. The more we keep doing things in this way, the pattern or "rut" become stronger. It takes about four to eight weeks for the imprint develop.

An example would be how you go to work every day. When you first started your job, you may have taken a certain route to work, until you found a quicker one with less traffic. Now that you have traveled that route countless times, there may be days when you get to work and don't even remember diving there. You were on auto pilot. That's a rut or a pattern in your brain. Your brain is "used to" that route so it doesn't really notice how you're getting to work.

So what does this mean? When it comes to chronic pain this means that the brain and the body are stuck in our holding patterns or this loop of constant pain. Even though the pain is not that bad anymore because it has healed, the pathway from the body to the brain is *saying that it is* because this pathway is the strongest. It was traveled for a long time, four to eight weeks, give or take, while the acute injury healed, or over years of holding and treating our bodies poorly.

Neuropathway: A neuropathway is a route that is followed by a nerve impulse that travels through either the central or peripheral nerve fibers of the central nervous system.

Here's a great way to visualize the neurons and neuropathways. Think of this pathway as the monorail at Epic Amusement World. The stops along the way where passengers get on and off are synapses—the junction between neurons. You get on this monorail and you see the excitement of your child (or adult) in anticipation of the day. With each stop more children and adults get on with excitement of the upcoming day. The excitement is almost infectious.

As these neurons (children) travel this pathway (monorail) they interact and give off signals (their excitement) to their surrounding neighbors (passengers) as they pass by. The signal that they produce has an effect on the surrounding neurons which continue traveling impacting the other interconnected neurons, continuing to relay information until the signal eventually reaches its intended target—the brain (Epic Amusement Park).

It can be as simple as a reflex, or a neuron arc (which is a pathway that a reflex travels), or it could be something that is a lot more complex. So if you think of your bad habits, they have become reflexes. We don't think about doing them because we have done them so often, we are on auto pilot.

We have learned from past experiences that certain things can harm us, help us, make us feel good, or make us feel terrible. From an early age our mothers tell us not to put our hands on the hot stove. How many of us actually had to touch it to find out she was right? Or, we listened but accidentally burnt our hands on a baking sheet? Our brains learned very quickly to be careful about making that same mistake. So we may lightly and quickly touch the pan or stove to double check to make sure it's not hot. Lorimer Moseley who is one of the world's leading experts on pain has an amazing way of explaining this on YouTube.

There are 16 areas of the brain that process pain. In nine of these areas, normally only five percent of the nerve cells are affected. But in those with chronic pain, a whopping 15 to 25 percent of these cells are affected. In a way, more cells were recruited for back up to help protect the body as this was a priority in keeping you safe. When the brain learns about the pain, like placing your hand on the hot stove, your brain protects the body by not touching it again, which is a good thing. But when these neuropathways become so strong and are traveled for so long, they go into overdrive or autopilot. The neurons become hypersensitive, typically due to a psychological or physical response. Then, in that hypersensitive mode, the feedback to the brain is misconstrued as being really bad, when it is not as the injury site has healed and it's really no longer that painful.

There was a television program called "Your Bleeped up Brain." I loved it. It would show different situations and request the viewer to pay attention to the man in the suit. Then after watching they would then replay it and look for other things. You as the viewer notice this giant gorilla in the background and you think, "How the hell did I miss that?!"

Or they would ask you to keep your eye on the magician and see if you can spot the red Ace. And after they ask you did you see it, it pointed out that while you were so diligently paying attention to the red Ace, the large painting in the background changed from blue to bright pink.

The amount of information that our brain processes at any given second is about 11,000,000 bits that it is receiving from the body. However, the conscious mind is really only able to process about 50 bits per second and has to decide in these split seconds how and what to do with this information

So you may be asking yourself, well how does the brain know what bits of information to process? The brain tends to process the strong and familiar ones.

Blazing New Trails in the Brain

Neuropathways that have been gone over and over again, like when your injury happened, have been traveled so often with the dimmer switch flipped to high beams, these pathways are like tire ruts in a dirt road. When you drive a truck down the same dirt rode two to five times a day, the ruts in the dirt become deeper.

The neuropathways that were created to warn the brain when your injury happened, have been traveled way more than two to five times a day. The dimmer switch was flipped to the ER bright (hypersensitive) setting numerous times from the injury site to the brain, and due to the frequency of their travel, they are now deeply engrained and now act like a default for the brain. The brain is used to receiving information from this pathway and figures that since it has been used so frequently in the last couple of months, it should probably keep paying attention to it. Especially since this pathway was established to protect you and keep you from creating further harm.

An example of a neuropathway less traveled would be when you hit your funny bone. More than likely you don't hit your funny bone very often. So, if you bump your elbow into a door, the dimmer switch will get flipped to high beams instantly and your brain is going to pay attention to it. Whacking your funny bone probably doesn't happen often and the alarm system isn't sounding frequently from this area. And because this does not happen often your brain is not going to pay it much attention once the pain decreases and you no longer hurt. The rut is not deep because you only drive down that road once or twice throughout the year.

The more often we perform the movement, the more natural it feels.

We see and feel this first hand when we practice yoga. In the beginning for those of us that have never done yoga or taken a yoga class, our first response is normally, "Oh hell no, that instructor has lost their mind thinking I'm going to be able to pull off that pose." We have just been asked to pull off the craziest crap ever. It scares us. But we attempt the pose and, in the beginning, our brain and our body are relaying information to each other trying to figure out what the hell is going on.

But once we start practicing yoga consistently, and do the pose over and over, the brain knows what the body is trying to, even though it may still think the body is crazy. And after a while many of the poses start to feel good and are no longer scary. In fact, they have a positive connotation connected to them!

But if we slightly turn our foot a different way, or interlace our fingers on the other side, this feels a little awkward. We are not used to doing the movements in this pattern because we haven't driven down this road often enough to have it feel familiar yet. But just in doing those simple movements we have created a new neuropathway. The more often we perform the movement, the more natural it feels.

If we look at it from the scientific point of view we are deviating from a set neuropathway of our current thinking and creating new neuropathways. This makes us smarter by weakening the current thought pattern that was traveled more often.

Each time we try a new pose and then repeat that pose in a future class, we are forcing our bodies to process the information of getting us into and out of that pose, making new neuropathways. One of the added benefits of yoga is that just about every time we do these yoga *asanas* (poses), we are challenging not only our bodies but our brains too become smarter.

It's easier for the brain to "assume" that it will receive this information on the roads that are traveled often because of how many bits of information it's receiving per second.

Let's just say that your injury was a knee injury that put you on this path of chronic pain. Think of a typical day running errands. Your brain is having to pay attention to you driving, and what the other cars are doing on the road.

Then it's focusing on you getting out of the car to run into the store to get the dry cleaning, and then back in the car, the kids are talking in the back seat, the phone is going off with a shit-ton of texts about don't forget the cupcakes, and you realize you need to get gas so you can go *back* and get the cupcakes and then take them to where they've got to be in the first place.

Your body is a magnificent, amazing, complex, efficient machine.

You park at the pump, get out of the car, you step slightly wrong on your leg while getting out of the car and, "Ouch! My knee!" You start to think, oh crap. It hurts. When in reality it doesn't really hurt. You're just uncomfortable. Your brain defaulted to "pain" because that is how strong that neuropathway was and how your brain is remembering the injury when it first happened, and the brain is not really paying attention to your pain because it's trying to remember where you left the damn cupcakes in the first place.

Your body is a magnificent, amazing, complex, efficient machine. We have protective mechanisms, the memories of how the injury took place as well as muscle spindles in our muscles that protect the body from going too far too soon to keep it safe. When we first get injured, our injured site sends off screaming warning signals o the brain saying, "Don't keep moving like that. You'll cause permeant damage if you do. We need to seek medical care right away." We need this so we do not continue to cause damage to that area.

However, after the acute injury has healed the neuropathway is strong and well-worn and is basically stuck in the "ER bright" position on the dimmer switch. When in reality when you got out of that car, your injured site was at the "sexy mood lighting" setting on the dimmer switch. But your brain was busy multitasking so it just "assumed" the injured site was in the "ER bright" position.

There are many new procedures that can be done and have had very good success in blocking the brain from staying in over drive. However, it still does not get to the underlying root cause of the problem. And just blocking the signals will only last for so long. Of course some people have better success than others with it.

If you are still doing and living in the same holding pattern (and I like to say holding pattern as this covers a lot of ground ... meaning your physical activity, how you hold yourself on a daily basis, your eating habits, your sleeping habits ... they all work together) you are not changing the neuropathway. You are still on the same strong chronic pain neuropathway when you need to be getting off that road and taking another.

But it's hard to get off a road you frequently travel and instead travel one that is unfamiliar. Especially if that road could potentially be seen as causing you more pain through movement and yoga. Just the thought of moving and trying to touch your toes gives you twinges of pain.

Hell, when you see those women stick their leg up behind their heads you feel pain. No way in hell you want to experience that! So, you limit your movements and you limit your activities. And I have to tell you, that's one of the worst things you can do for yourself.

It simply means that in order to break our bad habits we need to create healthier, happier habits. We can do this by changing our behavior which leads to new neuropathways. Neuropathways are the "train tracks" of our thought patterns and how we do things. When we live our lives, we continue to go down these pathways that feel comfortable and safe to us. We stay in these lanes because this is what we know. Going "outside the box" and down a dark alley can be scary. And as humans we like comfort—mental, physical and emotional. So we stay where we know what is going on and what is coming. Even if it's bad. The more we repeat these actions, behaviors and thoughts, the stronger become— which makes breaking them even harder!

So then the question becomes, how we can change these neuropathways? There are many ways. We can change them by our thoughts, soothing our emotions, images, sensations, beliefs and MOVEMENT. Yoga addresses all of these.

In the next chapter I'll give you better insight as to how practicing yoga can address your existing neuropathways and the ways yoga can help change your brain.

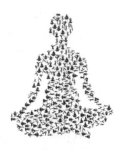

The quieter you become,
the more you can hear.
–Baba Ram Dass

***

Many of us are afraid of the quiet
because we are afraid of
what we will hear.
–Sam

5

This is Your Brain on Yoga

When we make a conscious effort to change a pattern or behavior, we then make a new neuropathway. We are not able to switch to this other neuropathway right away—that would be like a train jumping the track trying to get to the other track to change our direction.

As we slowly start to switch the strength of which this pathway is traveled, like a train track being re-routed, we may miss pulling the switch to change the direction of the tracks the first time. But as we come back around the next time, we'll be more aware we need to flip the switch. The more we travel this new neuropathway—the train track—it becomes more familiar to us through repetition, and we end up getting the timing down to just the right time to switch the train track and make a smooth transition.

In yoga we are able to soothe our emotions through the breath and though movement.

Becoming aware of how we are moving our bodies and when we are moving out bodies requires us to be mindful of what it is doing. It requires practice to get the timing of when to flip the track switch. Practicing yoga, we can do this.

In yoga we are able to soothe our emotions through the breath and though movement. The deep diaphragmatic breathing that we learn helps to stimulate the vagus nerve which helps to override our sympathetic nervous system—our fight or flight response. The sympathetic nervous system helps us run from the danger giving us with a ton of adrenaline which is a stress hormone. If you have ever been scared I'm sure you have found yourself either jumping and running in the opposite direction or stood your ground ready for what was coming around the corner ready to punch the crap out of it.

It Takes a Lot of Nerve

The vagus nerve plays a major role in our autonomic nervous system which controls the bodily functions that we do not think about like our breathing, our heartbeat and our digestive system. It is also the longest cranial nerve and contains motor and sensory fibers. And I'm sure you are asking by now, why the hell should I care? I'm so glad you asked.

The vagus nerve starts at the base of your brain, passes through your neck and ends in your abdomen. And where is your diaphragm located? The abdomen. When you take these deep diaphragmatic breaths doing yoga, you stimulate your vagus nerve.

When the vagus nerve is stimulated it relays the information up to the brain at a faster speed. So, when you are in stressful situations your sympathetic nervous system is in overdrive. Your brain is trying to decide whether you should be prepared to run from the clown because they are carrying a knife or stand your ground because they are going to make you a balloon animal. When the brain is able to receive this information about your environment and your current situation more quickly, your brain can make a better-informed decision.

Think of the vagus nerve like the Ice Train in Europe or the bullet trains in Asia. These trains are going to get you to our destination in two hours instead of five. The other trains will get you there, but they are going to stop off at every little town or village along the way. Just like your brain will receive the information your body is putting out, it's just going to take longer to get there.

When we stimulate our vagus nerve this stimulates the parasympathetic nervous system which is our feel-good system. You may have heard it called the feed or breed system. The parasympathetic system helps us to relax as well as conserves our energy, lowers our heart rate, and just makes us overall feel good.

When we practice yoga, the deep diaphragmatic breath stimulates the vagus nerve helping us to feel good, and the movement helps to simulate and release endorphins. I'm sure that you have heard of a "runner's high" which the person feels reduced anxiety and even feels less pain when they hit this "high". The runner feels they could keep running forever and they feel great. This is due mostly to the increase of endorphins surging throughout the brain. Our feel-good chemicals.

Endorphins are natural painkiller protein molecules that bind to receptors in the brain and spinal cord to help stop pain messages. Beta-endorphins in particular produce analgesia, which helps us to not feel pain, and then bind and interact with opioid receptors (these also help to block pain) and reduce our *perception* of pain.

In other words, these endorphins help to soothe our emotions which may be heightened by our pain or in anticipation of potential pain.

Thoughts Really Do Count

When we are experiencing chronic pain, we may feel anxious, depressed, sad, frustrated, etc. or a mix of these emotions at the same time. Anxious in anticipation if our back will lock up or if we'll be able to function to get out children to an important event. Depressed because we limit what we want to participate in for fear that we will trigger a migraine. Sad because we are not able to function and live how we would like. And frustrated that we are limited in what we are able to do.

Your thoughts actually have a positive or negative impact on a cellular level throughout your body. Remember how I explained that single neurons may not have much of an impact by themselves? But when a single positive neuron continues on the pathway it passes along its positivity to the other neurons it comes in contact with. There are some many books out there on positive thinking for a reason.

Same thing when we feel bad we tend to have negative thoughts (a negative neuron) which then lead to even more intense pain. When we feel good we tend to look at things from a better vantage point. We feel happier, we can change our perspective to more a positive one and that helps us to view our chronic pain as not being tolerable. You may feel that it's not so bad today. With this positive feeling you are also giving yourself hope that you can manage your pain, there is hope it may go away soon after all.

Positive thoughts have a direct impact on how we feel physically. Think about it. If you are feeling good, what do you do? You probably go for a walk or exercise, visit with family and friends, or eat a healthier meal. When we are in a happier mental state, we tend to make healthier lifestyle choices which leads our bodies to feel healthier. When we feel better about ourselves, physically and emotionally, the cycle of feeling good just continues. Endorphins, which come from movement and exercise, start to take effect and our perception of our pain shifts (remember I mentioned analgesia, and opioid receptors?) One reason why self-help books encourage you to say or think positive thoughts even if you don't feel like it.

The way we look at situations that arise throughout our day, positive or negative, has a direct correlation on how we feel and perceive our chronic pain.

As we continue making happier healthier choices we are changing the pattern and strength of our neurons. We are filling in the dirt rut of negativity and pain and replacing it with positive experiences and emotions. Happier healthy neurons equal new happy healthy neuropathways. And as we continue to choose to make healthier choices, we continue to increase our feel-good chemicals making us want more. The pathway (dirt rut) or unpleasant memory associated with your pain) that was once filled with pain and negativity, is now becoming filled with gold (or at least a bit of hope and a positive new memory).

Now, if you have ever experienced the shitty day at work, the boss didn't like the proposal that you spent all of your time and energy on, or the big meeting didn't deliver the results you were hoping for, you start to get in your head and become a bit depressed. Then what do you tend to want to do? Grab a drink, eat a pizza, candy and go home to sit on the couch and watch the newest episode of your favorite TV show. All you want to do is just lay there and go to bed. You feel crummy and if you have chronic pain, it may be much more noticeable to you. This gets makes getting out of bed even harder the next morning and the negative emotions and thoughts are with you the moment you open your eyes the next morning.

If you pause for a brief moment and think back to the positive paragraphs and this shorter negative paragraph, do you notice anything about how you feel?

The way we look at situations that arise throughout our day, positive or negative, has a direct correlation on how we feel and perceive our chronic pain. And the more we stay in a pattern of either being optimistic or a pessimist, these neuropathways become stronger and stronger. Whichever one it is.

In yoga we use a *mantra* which is the Sanskrit word for a word or sound repeated to help with concentration for meditation. For me this can be any positive word or thought, phrase or even an idea that helps me feel good about myself, my decisions and actions, or how to achieve my goals. When you silently or verbally repeat these mantras that are typically done and aid in meditation this repeated thought is forming a new connection affecting a nerve, neuron, or the nervous system which travels throughout your body. A neuropathway.

A mantra is a positive thought you keep going over so throughout your day it manifests (becomes) a positive reflex, whether that is how you respond to a situation or perform a task. You're planting your own seed in choosing good decisions and looking at things from a different positive perspective.

The Amazing Power of Music

The music that we listen to in yoga has a dramatic impact on our emotional state as well. Think about all of the types of music that you listen to and when you listen to it. How do you feel before and then after? Music plays a role in how our brains are processing information. Dance music comes on and you want to twerk. It helps you to feel happy and makes you just want to move. You may listen to jazz or piano music to help soothe and clam you after a long day at work. Or if you listen to rock it helps to pump you up so you can lift heavy in your weight lifting session. Music helps us to find states of calm, energy, or active pleasant memories. They call it "Baby making music" for a reason.

Research has shown these rhythmic signals and vibrations in music, can be beneficial in producing functional change when used in motor therapy for diseases such as Parkinson's disease, traumatic brain injury, strokes and many others. The rhythm in the music helps improve gait and upper extremity function in particular. The music directly impacts cognitive function, spatiotemporal reasoning attention as well as auditory verbal memory. (There's that memory things again.)

I want you to think of a negative experience. A negative memory. Close your eyes and notice how you feel. If you have seen someone get injured on a video have you felt your body physically react when you saw it happen? Or maybe you hear the sound of a car crash. You experienced no pain, yet your body responded out of the thought of it happening to you.

The memory of events can actually stimulate a physical reaction. If you close your eyes and think of a positive memory in a safe, warm, calming place or situation say the beach or doing something you really love that makes you happy, how do you physically feel? What do you remember hearing? Waves crashing onto the shore? The sound of laughter? Thinking of these situations and sounds do you find a smile spreading across your lips? I hope so.

A 16-year old student performed a simple experiment in 1997. It was supposed to see if music had an impact on cognitive function. He split the mice into three different groups and played different music to them for a week. One group got Mozart, one group got Anthrax the heavy metal group, and the other got no music. He had them do three runs through mazes and timed them.

In the beginning all the mice took an average of ten minutes to get through the maze. But by the end of the study, the mice who had no music cut their time by half to five minutes. No surprise, as they learned the maze. The Mozart mice remarkably finished the maze in an average time of a minute and a half! The Anthrax mice seemed to be drunk, banging into the walls, and now needed about 30 minutes to get through the maze. The crazy thing, this experiment was actually his second attempt. The first attempt he had to stop it early because he did not separate the mice and kept them all together in their groups. The reason this was a problem was the mice that were exposed to the Anthrax heavy metal became so aggressive that they bit each other to death until one lone mouse was standing.

A similar study used plants as its subjects. The plants that were played classical music grew towards the sound. Plants who were played death metal grew away from the sound. Another study found that vibrations from sound helped to stimulate cellular growth and boost immunity pathogens.

This is why specific chants and sounds are made during more traditional yoga classes. The sounds help to stimulate the brain as well as the vagus nerve, and other sensory nerves throughout the body. Especially in the CNS. The vibration helps to calm the CNS. There is a lot of research as well with yoga chants and the impact of helping slow Alzheimer's disease helping to improve memory.

So, if music can have that type of impact on creatures and vegetation, you would think that it would have an even greater impact on a human.

The imagery at the end of yoga in *savasana* (corpse pose or nap time) helps us to reinforce the thought patterns and new neuropathways we have been creating. Thinking of places, people or images or situations that help to calm us or bring us joy not only makes the brain healthy, but the physical body as well.

Throughout the yoga practice you were contracting your muscles making them stronger and increasing your flexibility. During this process you were creating small micro tears in your tissue. When done safely this is a great thing! When these small tears happen, this is when collagen can come in and repair the tissue making it stronger and bigger. Then in *savasana*, you are able to allow the physical tension to release. Being mindful of a specific area then making a choice, taking action and allowing that area to relax.

When we are more aware of the positive sensations and the actions that we took or need to take to recreate these sensations, we reinforce the new neuropathways (memories) that we created.

You are basically replacing the old negative neuropathway (memory) that was associated with movement and are replacing it with a positive neuropathway (memory). One that you'll want to revisit.

If you encounter a yoga class that incorporates essential oils these smells directly impact our brains by stimulating the amygdala—the area of the brain that deals with pain, emotion, emotional memory, sight, pleasure, smell and other sensations. When the holidays come around you light certain scented candles. These candles and scents that you choose give you feel-good feeling or bring back positive memories. When you think of this memory it may make you smile and feel good. Typically, people don't want to have a bad memory or smell something like rotten fish or crap. The first thing you reflexively do is scrunch up your nose and curly a lip and take a step back. Your body physically tenses with such a smell. All of these senses, emotions, memories, movements and beliefs are all controlled by the main hard drive, the brain.

In the beginning when you do start moving and really becoming physically active again, you will experience some discomfort. Your brain may want to perceive it as pain, but you'll actually only be a bit uncomfortable. I am not saying that you will never experience some pain as you progress in your movement and yoga practice, but I will provide you with some guidelines in Chapter 10 to help keep yourself safe as you start moving again. But until we get to that Chapter 10, I want to go over reasons you will or may experience discomfort.

Many times when you start moving after your doctor has told you are allowed to resume to previous activities, the discomfort you feel first is contributed to a hypersensitivity in your fascia. Keep reading and I will explain.

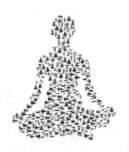

Around here, we don't look
backwards for very long ...
we keep moving forward,
opening up new doors
and doing new things
because we're curious,
and curiosity keeps leading
us down new paths.

—Walt Disney

6

Fascia Fitness and Hypersensitivity

I'm sure you have heard of it. It's all the rage these days: "Blast through your cellulite with fascia fat blasting tools and alleviate your pain!!!"

I'm sure you may have come across an ad for this on your favorite social media thread. These techniques *do* work. They do help alleviate the pain short term. But I also feel that this is the lazy way out. If you are only using these types of surface manipulation tools, the likelihood of decreasing your pain long-term is very small.

I believe that if you use tools like a foam roller *in conjunction with* yoga and other tools and modalities like acupuncture and massage therapy, you can create your perfect "holistic" cocktail to combating your chronic pain and taking back control of your life.

Remember what I said earlier? There is no magic pill, or physical exercise, or diet, or pillow. Everyone is different and will respond differently to different techniques. The magic pill is YOU!

There's no doubt that fascia does play a role in your movement and chronic pain. Now the question becomes, do you really understand what your fascia is and why it's important to become educated about it? NO? Well you are in luck. In this chapter I'll breakdown what fascia is, what it does and why you should care.

Fascia—It's Not Just a Fad

Fascia is a fibrous connective tissue found all throughout your body. In recent years we've learned so much more about how extensively our fascia is intertwined throughout our bodies than originally thought.

There are three different kinds of fascia:

1. Superficial fascia—primarily found around your skin.

2. Deep fascia—typically found adjacent to your muscles, bones, nerves and even your blood vessels.

3. Visceral fascia—found near the organs.

These tissues are designed to move and glide over each other with ease and little effort. You can think of fascia as an internal girdle for your organs, skeletal structure, muscles ligaments and tendons. Fascia also acts as a "safety net" or a sponge to help keep fluid near all of these. Why is fluid important? The average human body is made up of roughly 60 percent water. The brain and the heart are composed of about 70 percent water; the lungs, 83 percent; skin, 64 percent; muscles and kidney, about 79 percent (give or take on all of these numbers). The importance of water is a HUGE game changer in your chronic pain. (I'll get into more of that later on as well.)

Over time, as movement declines, the fascia becomes denser and it's more painful as we break through the sensitive fascia when we get moving again.

If you have ever prepped a turkey or chicken ready for roasting and pulled up the skin, you slide your hand between the skin and the meat to put butter or other herbs and seasoning on to get ready to cook. That thin layer of "webbing" that you easily swiped away is an example of fascia of the animal.

If you are like me, and not a chef, here is another way of looking at it.

Think of a Spiderman suit or fishnet stockings. If you have ever seen a spiderweb that has just been started and a gust of wind comes along it just *poof!* ... disappears. If you come across a spiderweb that has been there for a while (or the cotton fake spiderwebbing you see around Halloween) a gust of wind comes long it may not disappear or it may end up clumps here and there. I am *not* saying that your fascia clumps, but this gives you a visual of how the fascia is supposed to work. Ideally, you are moving enough throughout your day that when you do move, the fascia stays flexible and pliable. When the fascia is not moved on a daily basis it can become fibrous and hard. Once you start moving that area it is going to be uncomfortable.

There are numerous fascia lines that run throughout the body. (My favorite reference on this topic is *Anatomy Trains* by Thomas Myers.) There are said to be 12 meridian fascial lines that travel throughout your body—on your sides, front and back. They go from one side of your body to the other. Then there's a line of fascia that goes all the way from the ball of your foot, up the back of your legs, up your back, and all the way up to your head.

Many of us tend to think inside the box and in a linear process. We forget about how our fascia and our kinetic chain are connected. When we know about these connections, it makes more sense that when we rub our feet, our headache seems to ease. (I'll explain more about the importance of the kinetic chain in Chapter 7.)

Every cell, every system and organ in your body is connected to the fascia.

An example is if your feet have been sore and you successfully talk your partner into giving you a foot rub, have you noticed how your whole body feels more relaxed? Once we gain a better understanding to how the fascia is connected throughout the entire body it's easier for us to understand why when our lower back hurts we get a headache. Or when you get that foot rub your headache eases.

These fascia lines are more of a stability system for your internal body. It connects to every organ and all of your muscles all the way from the bottom of your feet to the top of your head. Every cell, every system and organ in your body is connected to the fascia. This is super cool to know because now we know that the way that we physically train, move, stretch and lengthen our body to lose weight or gain muscle mass we can alter the way our bodies feel and function by basically restructuring (remolding) our fascia. We can get the cells in your body to actually change their function. It's a radical new way of seeing personal training-stretching, strengthening and shape-shifting-as part of "spatial medicine."

For those that do resistance training, we lift to build muscle. Some do it as a hobby and to compete in bodybuilding competitions. Some do resistance training so their butts will look good in their jeans. If those reasons do not sound appealing to you, look at it this way. It is common for women as we age to have early stages of osteoporosis due to calcium depletion through the joys of being a woman. One of the most important reasons to lift weights and do resistance training is to help support our skeletal structure. For women as we age it is extremely important to have strong muscles to support our bones. Research has proven that one of the most effective ways to increase bone density is weight bearing exercise.

When we change the shape and the strength of our muscles, the fascia changes as well. The fascia molds around the muscles and helps to give support and shape to our bodies. The fascia helps to hold the bones together by compressing the muscles tighter to the skeletal system. Kind of like a girdle for your insides which will also help you look great for that skin-tight dress.

The more muscle mass you have the denser the muscle becomes. The muscle will start to grow and gain in size and in way start to push outward. This is why you are able to see muscle definition so well as you increase your muscle mass. The fascia helps to support the muscle providing a smoother shape. As you lift weights the muscle mass you build is a "side effect" to the exercise. I like that kind of side effect. The fascia will reshape itself and conform to the muscles as they reshape and grow. This can happen from direct cellular signaling. This really just means that one cell is getting direct interaction from a neighboring cell or from the action of that cell. If one cell is changing shape, the nearby cell will change shape too. You can think of it as peer pressure from its nearby associates. They just want to fit in, so they change too.

Reshaping Your Fascia

Some of the ways to help restructure your fascia are by foam rolling, Rolfing (a style of massage), resistance training and you guessed it ... yoga!

One of the best things you can do for your fascia is to move. Movement, pressure, loading the tissue as well as friction are ways you are able to keep the fascia soft and pliable. You need your fascia to move. Not so much to where it allows the tissues or bones that it is supporting to move. You don't want your nerves having free reign to go and explore from your spine. But you need it to be fit to move enough to allow the joints and tissues it is supporting to function how they need to. Your fascia also has to have some movement to help fluid flow throughout your body. Water and other fluids help to nourish and hydrate the tissues and organs.

If you tell some individuals they need to stretch to move their fascia they may take it to the extreme with the thought if they can stretch it really quick they will get results faster.

Not so with the fascia. The American want of instant gratification is denied again.

After an accident, surgery or lack of movement for long periods of time, you will need to get the fascia to lengthen and become supple again. But in order to do this correctly it will require some pressure, time, gentle movement and tension that is applied over long periods of time that seem to work the best. And guess what activity does that throughout your entire body? You guessed it ... yoga.

We are continuing to learn every day something new about the fascia, so this information may change. The fact that yoga is good for you won't. When you change the demand on the muscles by overloading them with more weight, changing the repetitions or sets, contorting your body into different yoga asanas, you are able to do the same thing with your fascia. Yoga poses, like spinal twists, not only help to massage your internal organs to help detoxify them and wake them up to get working like they are intended to, but these poses also help to get to the deep fascia that encompasses your organs and to get your deep visceral fascia.

Another great thing about yoga is that you are able to reach the end range of the muscles to create strength and flexibility. When I say end range, I am referring to being able to access the entire muscle. Depending on who you talk to, there are many different thoughts when it comes to stretching and flexibility. Research is varying and has been for years on the topic of stretching and I'm sure it will continue to be for a while. Some think that too much flexibility is a bad thing, which it is. Hypermobility can be very problematic for some. But I personally think that the majority of the population will benefit from stretching, lengthening and increasing flexibility in their muscles.

If your body has more flexibility ...
you are better prepared for when life happens.

Here's my logic. When you're not moving and exercising regularly, your muscles get tight. If your muscles are tight, your muscles are weak. There is no such thing as a strong tight muscle.

Think of it this way. If your hamstring is 20 inches long (I just picked a number out of the air) and if your hamstrings are so tight you are only able to use 12 inches of that muscle, you are missing out on eight more inches of strength potential. With yoga, however, you are able to increase your odds of getting to that end range of the muscles—that entire 20 inches—to create strength and flexibility.

The reason why this is important is that with tight, shortened muscles you are limiting the power that you can use in your golf swing, your vertical jump, your pitch and how efficiently your body can move and function throughout the day. Tight muscles limit your walking gait and can alter your foot striking patterns. If you have greater range of motion in your muscles, and they are stronger, they will be able to adapt and help you when life happens.

What I mean is if you are training for a 5k run, you might end up just rolling—instead of breaking—your ankle because you accidently stepped off the curb wrong, or stepped in a pothole while you were running. Or in the winter when you accidently step and slip on black ice. If your body has more flexibility and greater range of motion, as you step out wide to catch yourself before falling, you are better prepared for when life happens. Your body can more easily adapt and protect itself.

Our bodies are going to be so much more willing to adjust and compensate for when life happens when our fascia is moving with more ease and is not contributing to limiting the way that our bodies move. We can look at this as even preventive injury medicine. The natural kind. At least this is how I like to look at it.

In yoga you constantly pay attention to your posture and the way you hold yourself during a class. You practice being mindful of how your body is reacting and responding to what you're doing at that moment. You're honing your spatial awareness, which means where your body is in space.

If you're in a balancing half-moon, or some other challenging balance pose, but not paying attention, the possibility of you falling over drastically increases. This wobbling in class can be attributed to the mind being focused on what you are going to make for dinner and/or it could be that your stabilizer muscles (which are the muscles that help to stabilize and steady you while the major muscles do the majority of the work) aren't strong yet.

What you are practicing throughout the yoga class translates into your daily life. When you practice holding yourself upright the way that your body is designed to be held, with proper taller posture and tight abdominal muscles so your pelvis is able to stay biomechanically positioned under your ribs where they are designed to be, your fascia starts to remold as well. It starts to support the muscles, skeleton and other tissues because of the way you are training them. As your fascia becomes healthier, you'll have better overall functional movement, potentially decreasing other types of injury, helping to catch small problems before they start to become bigger ones (like holding yourself in a poor posture). And, our butts will look tighter and great in our jeans. That's what I call a win win.

Is It Stretching, or Yoga?

What I've learned throughout the 15 years I have been teaching yoga, is that depending on your audience, the buy in as to why you should do yoga varies.

I personally don't care what people call it, as long as they keep moving.

For the Special Forces Operators I worked with, the total bad asses of the military, (thank you to all) we called it stretching. When I first started working with them I would ask how many of them had ever done yoga. A few would raise their hands. As I started to show them basic yoga flows such as a sun salutation I would typically hear, "Hey, I've done this stretch before." Which I then replied, "See. You have done yoga. Yoga has been around longer than the word stretches has existed. But we'll just keep calling it stretching so we don't accidently scare your testosterone."

It's all about perspective. I personally don't care what people call it, as long as they keep moving. A burpee is a moving sun salutation in my opinion.

Yin yoga is a style of yoga in where you hold the poses, asanas, for long periods of time, three to five minutes. These days this type of yoga is called "static stretching" so men can feel "macho" about yoga. Most people cannot stand this type of yoga class. They find it boring and uncomfortable. But, its systematic approach is extremely beneficial in creating strong, flexible muscles than "stretching" after a workout.

What do you typically see at the gym after a workout? If it was arm day, maybe okay let's stretch the biceps ... got it ... now on to the triceps .... It's just a few seconds each and just a thrown-in afterthought of random—frankly, half-assed— stretches. It's not giving the muscles all the benefits that deep, long stretching does, nor does such mindless "stretching" help the muscles heal.

Depending on what research study you read, they say that there really is no added benefit from holding a stretch longer than a minute, and especially no longer than three minutes. I disagree. Why? Here's my thought process. Let me give you an example of a typical yoga pose for someone with chronic pain. For this example, my magic number is a three-minute stretch. (If Yin yoga holds poses for three to five minutes, and Western researchers are saying there's no added benefit especially after three minutes, I'll go with the common denominator which is the number three.)

For those that have chronic pain, for the first minute of a pose, they are so uncomfortable they are just trying to gain control of their breath and figure out how to ease into the pose. I have seen it time and time again as those who have severe chronic pain keep moving around trying to get comfortable and just the right way to position their body.

After that first minute they are able to find a way to get into the pose and start to relax, the second minute they pretty much just getting through the superficial layer of fascia, which can be very hypersensitive (i.e. where the "pain" is coming from—I'll talk more about this later). And then the third minute as the relaxation deepens, you can get to more of the meat and potatoes of the body ... the deepest fascia, muscles, ligaments, tendons and organs.

Granted this is just my hypothesis and my thought process. (Like I said in the Introduction, I have a lot of opinions.)

The same concept is true for increasing the flexibility in your muscles. Some believe[2] that a muscle really only has about four to eight percent range of motion to stretch in a safe manner. If you stretch safely and efficiently you will create these little micro tears and lay down collagen to build up healthier stronger muscles. But if you go too far past a muscle's range of motion before it's ready, that is when you pull, tear, or rip the muscle. Now you are laying down scar tissue which will never be 100 percent healthy again. Just another reason to take things slow. (Reminder: The tortoise always wins!)

Now when it comes to your chronic pain, let's say from an injury you sustained, more than likely your physician recommended that you wait four to eight weeks for this acute injury to heal well enough to get back to normal activity. In this amount of time you may have gotten into the habit of guarding and limiting your movements in your daily activities and unconsciously protecting yourself. Possibly even having to give up your regular workout routines. (For some of us this lack of movement is torture!) But this lack of movement is a normal and natural way that the body protects itself from further harm and helps us heal.

The problem that is brewing under the surface in this time frame, is with limited movement and restricting your natural movement patterns, the fascia basically becomes thicker and thicker and more rigid. Remember how I mentioned that your fascia helps to keep fluid around the tissues? Well, if the fascia has limited movement it is not as effective as keeping or moving fluids throughout the body. In a way it kind of sticks together. With daily movement and exercise—even if it was just putting away the dishes, or throwing a load of laundry in the washer— you were moving and keeping this fascia from getting stuck.

This is a main reason why you are so sore and in "pain.".

The reason why this lack of movement, and how it plays into your chronic pain and your yoga practice, is important is because as I said earlier, pretty much just about every cell is connected into this fascia web. They have found that your fascia has more than *ten times more sensory nerve endings* than anywhere else in your body. This is a main reason why you are so sore and in "pain."

When you start to get this fascia "unstuck" and moving again after your injury has healed, many times this is what is really making you uncomfortable. It is normally *not* the injury that you initially had because that has healed in those four to eight weeks. The discomfort you are actually feeling is coming from creating small micro tears in the fascia when you start to get your fascia "unstuck." When you do this this safely, you will be uncomfortable but you are not doing any harm to your body. This hypersensitivity plays a huge role in your chronic pain.

Why? As you move on a daily basis you are constantly stimulating these sensory nerves, and this becomes their norm. When you move around and go through your daily activities and fitness programs you keep yourself desensitized. Movement in general helps to keep you desensitized through the constant stimulation these nerves are receiving. Movement creates sensation, sensation helps to keep you desensitized. When the sensory nerves are used to this movement they know that you are not hurting them, so there is no cause for alarm.

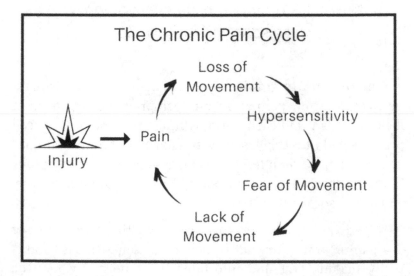

The less active you are, the more sensitive you become because you are no longer stimulating these sensory nerves as often as you typically do. So when you do start moving again, starting to move your fascia again can be extremely uncomfortable. You may think it's your muscles, ligaments, or other body parts, or the injury that you sustained that is causing you this "pain," but more than likely it's your fascia that you are first feeling the "pain" or discomfort in. With increased "pain" and discomfort comes even move limited movement and activity because we perceive this as pain and we think back to the memory of our injury.

This hypersensitivity is a small portion of why you have chronic pain. It is a symptom/side effect of a bigger picture.

An easy example of this hypersensitivity is after the winter is over and spring and summer start to become ever so inviting, you find yourself being a little less careful about putting shoes on before going outside to check the mail. Or you gravitate towards the patio furniture or hammock on a warm day. At first your feet may feel every little pebble, rock, brick, or stick that you come across as you make your way across the yard. But towards the end of the summer, these small little rocks that you were so aware of earlier in the season you hardly seem to notice as you run after your kids in the yard. You have desensitized your feet and are aware that you are not in danger.

The same thing happens when you move around going through your daily activities, doing the laundry, bending over to clean the floors, walking up stairs and other physical activities you partake in. You keep yourself desensitized in this daily movement.

If you have ever been kicking ass in the gym to get ready for that new bikini, you were probably working hard, sore as hell but wanting to accomplish that bod you so desperately desired. And once you hit your goal, and were rocking that bikini, you told yourself that you were going to have fun, take it easy, and did not end up going to the hotel fitness center because you deserved a break.

When you come back to reality from your vacation and hit the gym because now you feel guilty putting back on those five pounds that you worked so desperately hard to get off in the first place, the same exercises and activities that you did before you went on vacation and didn't seem to bother you, holy crap you are definitely aware of that soreness now! In this short amount of time you were on vacation, you became more sensitive. Daily activity and movement helps to keep you desensitized.

Individuals who have this hypersensitivity start to feel that it takes longer for their pain to disappear or to fade. Once again, this hypersensitivity is not the reason why you have chronic pain; it is just a symptom of multiple factors. One of which is how your brain perceives pain—that's neuroplasticity.

As your movement has been restricted while your injury was healing, your neuropathways were on heightened alert, receiving warning signals from the injured area for the last four to eight weeks continuing to protect you so you are able to heal and get better. This lack of movement, which has led to a hypersensitivity and the constant warnings, has thrown your CNS (central nervous system) out of whack (as mentioned in Chapter 4).

This lack of movement then keeps your fascia from moving the way that it is designed to as well as keeping the CNS desensitized. When you start to move and are hypersensitive, this feeds into the kinesiophobia that leads to catastrophizing as well as avoidance continuing your chronic pain cycle.

So then the question becomes ... how the hell do you not feed into this fear? I'm so glad you asked. We'll dive into the fear-movement cycle in Chapter 8, but first, there's there is a stop on this tour of the miraculous human body that needs to be visited: the kinetic chain.

As you continue on to the next chapter, you'll learn more about how the body is connected and the importance of your hips. Yup, your hips. The middle ground and gate keeper to the Utopia of a pain free life. (Utopia: an *imagined* place or state of things in which everything is perfect).

You notice the word imagine is italicized? Friendly reminder ... You are not entitled to a pain free life. A pain free life does not exist. If you are living life, you will experience some type of pain at some point. But understanding how your hips can help to diminish or intensive or create your chronic pain getting to point A to point B as you are living, helps.

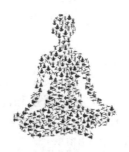

*When life gets you down,
you know what you gotta do?
Just keep swimming!*

–Dory, *Finding Nemo*

7

The Kinetic Chain: The Hips Don't Lie

Human anatomy has been absolutely fascinating to me, pretty much for my whole life. I find it so interesting how the simple rotation of a palm, or the turnout of a foot can change the way a muscle or group of muscles work.

I understand how for some it may not be the least intriguing to them because all they think of is the how they are not able to sit down on a toilet after a killer leg day.

It can be a bit confusing and complicated, especially with medical and anatomy talk. But having a good basic simple understanding of how your body relates and reacts to itself is important on gaining control of your chronic pain and applying it to your yoga practice.

Some of what we've discussed—like the central nervous system—might ring some bells from high school biology. Other topics, like fascia, may be fairly common to you these days. In this chapter, we'll wrap up our trip down Anatomy Lane with a look at the Kinetic Chain (and, no, it's not a new PlayStation game or a piece of jewelry).

It's All Connected

The simple explanation of the kinetic chain is that our body is a series of overlapping muscles, segments and joints that affects other joints and muscles that in turn allow effective and efficient movement. When one muscle moves and is in motion, it creates a chain of movement from other nearby joints and muscles—kind of like a domino effect.

When people sustain an injury or have lower back pain, they many times forget that their whole body is connected and intertwined. If they have an injury or a flare up, that problem area is many times the main focus all of their energy because that is the "source" of their discomfort. Totally understandable.

However, there are many times where the area of the body that is flared up and sore is actually the end result of another problem elsewhere in the body. There are times the injured area is truly flared up and pissed off, and many times this flare up could have been prevented if other issues throughout your body had been addressed. There is a possibility that these other areas of the body may be causing the flare up or at least contributing to the problem.

Relating this to your chronic pain, if you have been dealing with your issue for months or years, more than likely the best minds in the medical field have tried to figure out what is wrong with you and still don't have an idea. Or if they know what your problem is and they can't "fix" you. In that case I guess you've been kind of screwed up till now.

So now it's time to take back control of the wheel and start steering the car the direction you want it to go. Remember how I mentioned the tachometer on the car? If you keep throttling on the gas, you'll blow your engine. If you leave the car on the side of the road in winter, you'll freeze and you'll be a bear's dinner.

Ask yourself where do you want to go? You have an open road in front of you and you get to travel wherever you want. Oh the possibilities!

Your Body's Chain Reaction

So here is a basic run down of your kinetic chain and why you need to pay attention to it.

Let's start at the pelvis. The pelvis is a large semicircular bone that forms the base on which the upper body is positioned. The pelvis was built to provide a foundation for other parts of the anatomy like the back and legs to connect to so you can move about this wonderful world. Your pelvis is the axis point, the middle ground of your body. It is the juncture of your upper body and lower body. Our quadriceps, hamstrings, piriformis, and hip flexors (and others that I like to throw into the pile known as "glutei meat") all attach to your pelvis. They help you move your leg forward, backward, and from side to side. They also help you to bend, sit, and stand and so on. The pelvis plays a huge role in our day-to-day function and movement.

You can head to YouTube to see some great videos with fantastic graphics that may explain it better.

What I want to do is to try to explain this in the simplest way possible to you. It is so important to open up our hips on a daily basis. We constantly use them throughout the day in walking, standing, going up the stairs, coming down the stairs, sitting, etc. But then how often do we give them TLC? Most of you will say, rarely if never.

Many people think that our pelvis and our hips are the same thing, but the hips are a joint that has four bones that form a ball and socket joint. The hip allows us to move and distribute the weight of our body throughout our legs and provides us with stability. The hip and the pelvis are connected to the femur by ligaments. The hip flexors, extensors, adductors, and external rotators basically allow us to have 360-degree range of motion. The hip flexors attach the lower part of the spine and pelvis, cross over the hip joint and then attach to the top of the femur (thigh bone).

So now, your body is fighting with itself over the pelvis.

Then we have our psoas major muscle, which connects to the T12 vertebra in your spine, wraps around the front of the pelvis, and then connects to the femur. The iliacus and the psoas combine to form one muscle known as the iliopsoas. If this muscle is tight—and many people have a tight psoas due to poor posture and being in "slump asana" all day. (A yoga teacher joke, this refers to being in that slumped-over, hunched-down position at your desk). We are constantly slumped over our computers, our steering wheel, our kids, etc. We constantly have our bodies working overtime to hold ourselves in a way that we are really not biomechanically designed to be in for long periods of time.

Now when this psoas muscle is tight, think of it like a rubber band, that wants to pull the pelvis towards your belly button. Your tight leg and glutei meat want the pelvis to tilt their way towards the thighs because those muscles are tight, and your back/torso wants your pelvis to tilt towards your chest. So now, your body is fighting with itself over the pelvis. And all the pelvis wants to do is have them both get along.

Now think of this. Now that your psoas has been fighting with our legs and glutei meat muscles all day, the other muscles in your back are working overtime to hold you in upright position all day trying to get you to sit and stand up straight. So now your lats, rhomboids, and trapezius muscles are pissed off, tired and fatigued because they have been trying to support your torso keeping you upright. They have been forced to over compensate and work harder to do someone else's job (the psoas) who has been trying to keep your pelvis biomechanically where it should be.

Think of a co-worker that is a bit lazier than you are. Or think of a friend or a loved one who has to work harder because their co-worker doesn't do their job. It's got to get done, so who picks up the slack? Same thing with your body.

Now that these back muscles are tight and pissed off then you start to get a headache. Many times this is because your trapezius muscles are tight which are in close proximity to your occipital belly which are close to your temporalis (which are located on your skull) and so on and so on. When the adjacent muscles are having to work harder at their job it's a chain reaction for the surrounding muscles to have to work harder as well.

The same thing with your legs. If your quadriceps, glutes, hamstrings are all tight, they are having to work harder to get you from point A to point B all day long: standing, sitting, squatting, walking, living. They get tight and fatigued. And if they're tight they are now limiting your natural range of motion and walking gait which once again requires the body to over compensate to hold and move you in a correct position that should be easy. But it's *not* easy because your body is fighting with itself (those tight muscles) and holding excessive loads of weight in ways that it is not designed to do.

This change in your walking and gait pattern then travels down your legs to your calves, ankles and feet. When your walking/gait pattern is off, this many times will cause your feet to strike in a way that it is not supposed to carry you. The weight of your body will cause the load on your feet to be distributed at odd angles and ways that the foot is not designed to function in. Possible foot conditions that can be associated with this is flat foot, or plantar fasciitis.

According to the Mayo Clinic, plantar fasciitis is one of the most comes causes for heel pain. It's common in runners, but also in people who are overweight. The plantar fascia is a shock absorbing bowstring that is located in the arch of your foot and if the load or tension that is being distributed on the arch is too great, small tears occur. Repetitive stretching and tears can cause it to inflame. Guess what helps with stretching your feet and ankles? Down dog. Yoga.

*The best-informed decision is not to stop moving.
It is to modify your movement.*

And then you ask yourself why your lower back hurts? To be honest I'd be surprised if it didn't hurt. It's not rocket science all. It's Newton's third law of motion. For every action, there is an equal and opposite reaction. This statement means that in every interaction, there is a pair of forces acting on the two interacting objects.

Why do car manufacturers spend millions of dollars in figuring out the best way to design cars and trucks the way they do? In order for you to pay a shit-ton of money to get the best possible truck or car that with provide you with the smoothest ride, be able to pull the heaviest load of bricks possible while going over all of those hills, dirt and creeks while off-roading so you won't feel a bump or pot hole while you work hard. (Once again, marketing is a great thing.)

Having this better understanding of your kinetic chain and how you are biomechanically designed will benefit you as you learn to modify, if needed, perform the yoga poses correctly to keep yourself safe, and/or why a yoga pose is agitating your medical issue. Just another step in gaining back control of your pain. Once you have a better understanding of what is possibly flaring up your issue, you are able to make a better-informed decision about how to correct it. Oh, and the best-informed decision is *not* to stop moving. It is to *modify* your movement.

Many times we just go through the moments and motions. "Feel your breath and connect it to the movement. Just flow." All well and good if you know how to do the *asana* correctly and if you are strong enough to do it correctly. But if you are new to yoga or have a medical issue, you could possibly be guarding yourself. Your brain in trying to protect the body unconsciously, so it does things and changes your movements based off of past experiences, memories or perceived pain that is no longer there or that you are experiencing. This relates to your neuroplasticity.

When your brain is trying to protect itself from injury, you might be moving or holding yourself in a position that is going to tick off and perturb the injured part without realizing it. It might feel good in the beginning but that is because your brain is getting a quick shot of feel good endorphins. It will feel good in the moment, but then later on as the day goes by your back seems to get worse. Kind of like not wearing a condom. It feels good at the time, but you many times end up having more complications from not wearing one.

I am not surprised when I hear this. (Not about the condoms, the endorphins.) We want to feel good. Many times to get that feeling of relaxation you allow your back to slump because it is fatigued. It's fatigued because you are not requiring or strengthening your back muscles to work and become strong to hold you in a tall posture all day. When you slump to allow your back muscles to relax you also stretch out your back muscles. These back muscles are deconditioned just like another muscle in your body. So when you do start becoming aware of keeping your posture nice and tall, your back gets tired.

When you slump, you may end up staying in that slumped position much longer than you should. When you stay in this slumped posture you end up holding your spine in a position where it is not in a neutral alignment and you overload your facet joints. These facet joints are located in your spine.

Pressure that is applied to these facet joints can be caused by several things, one of which is just the simple fact that as we age in intervertebral discs in your spine degenerate. When the discs start to degenerate and wear down this can lead to narrowing of the space between the vertebrae which then affects the way that the facet joints line up. If this occurs, it places too much pressure on the articular cartilage surface of the facet joint and eventually the cartilage begins to wear away.

The intervertebral discs are a made out of lamellae, which are concentric sheets of collagen fiber, and connect to the vertebral end plates. They are located in between the spinal vertebrae and act as a shock absorber and help facilitate movement without grinding your boney vertebra against each other. There is also a possibility depending on the severity of the bulging disc could leave to impingement on the surrounding nerves as well.

If you have been informed that you have a bulging disc, approximately 90 percent of bulging discs typically happen in your lower back, the disc has basically shifted outside of its "normal" position in between the vertebrae. This can happen with multiple different physically stressors. And is very common. So when you slump and if you have a bulging disc that has been slightly misplaced, the possibility of disc being pinched by the spinal vertebrae is much greater. A pinched disc can cause intense pain and discomfort. But there are MANY that go their whole lives with bulging discs with no symptoms and pain what so ever.

Finding Freedom in Structure

You and your doctor are right. You need to go take a yoga class. But when you do finally drag your ass to one, the instructor leads you through a series of movements and postures that your body is not structurally designed to carry and to do at this moment with the extra weight that is having to bear. Then you end up ticking off the body part or medical issue and you swear off yoga and never go back. Oh yeah ... I've heard that a hundred times too.

Don't get me wrong. You want to move your body and especially your spine. We need it and want it to extend, twist, and bend, but just not in ways that is going to compromise it. And there is a difference between rounding and extending your spine in a safe slow controlled manner, and then staying in a fixed position which pinches the discs causing inflammation and irritation.

I love the saying, "Yoga is not about touching your toes, it's about the journey on the way down." To have people hold their bodies or to have their students go from a forward fold to a standing position and cuing, "Imagine slowly stacking our vertebra on top of each other one at a time until you come to mountain pose" can create discomfort and irritation by pinching the discs and pissing of the back or neck. I don't recommend it.

The problem comes into play when these patients walk into the yoga boutique studio on the corner and that instructor doesn't really understand their medical condition.

There are ways of being able to move the spine and sequence it to be beneficial and help instead of jacking yourself up more, so many times when an instructor cues this, they should not be. (My own personal opinion and advice to those with back problems. Take it or leave it. The choice is yours.) This is how I know this.

In my previous job, I was one the first permanent chronic pain trained yoga therapists in one of the Army's new chronic pain movement recovery programs. I was tasked with using holistic approaches to combating chronic pain to help reduce the use of prescription opioid medications and to provide patients with ways of dealing with their chronic pain and get them moving again.

Many providers understand and believe that yoga is good for the patient and can be very beneficial. I know many providers that recommend their patients to take yoga classes.

The problem comes into play when these patients walk into the yoga boutique studio on the corner and that instructor doesn't really understand their medical condition or have a good way or idea in how to help them modify for their particular issue.

I have had many of the physicians that I worked with come and take my classes. In particular I had an anesthesiologist that came and took a couple of my classes to have a better idea of what and how I was working with the patients. In one of the sessions he informed me that he had chronic lower back pain. He started doing yoga at a local boutique yoga studio at his previous duty location. He did yoga for two years and his back seemed to get worse. But they told him to keep doing yoga and it will get better. It didn't.

In taking him through a simple sun salutation, in the first forward fold, the cobra and his down dog, I found several things that I could see would lead to his back pain. I instructed him how to modify the poses so it did not agitate his back, and then what do you know ... it helped! He then looked at me and said, "So why did nobody tell me how to modify these poses before? My back already feels better with these modifications." Because those instructors did not know.

It's Not All the Instructor's Fault

The world is full of yoga instructors. Some that are amazing, some that are good. Some that are fresh out of school. All, I believe, have good intent. Yet not every yoga instructor is created equal. Many out there give cues throughout a class that aggravate and inflame your existing condition.

Yoga instructors just like many other teachers teach what and how they were taught. There are many instructors are trained in more "traditional" forms of yoga practices from India. These traditional forms of practice work for a population that is genetically inclined to be able to perform these poses, who do not have many medical issues, and where it's their culture to start practicing it from a young age.

Moreover, many of these yoga poses are going to be challenging for men and then some for women due to our genetic make-up. You do not need to be a medical provider to know that a woman's body is definitely not biomechanically designed like a man's. (Thank goodness or babies would be an even bigger bitch to push out.)

Also, something I noticed, it could be something or it may not be anything at all, if you watch Indian men ride on bicycles, their hips and legs seem to externally rotate more naturally. This is genetically different than the typical male in the United Sates.

The key is finding what style of yoga will benefit you.

Still, a number of yoga instructors gravitate toward more traditional Eastern yoga poses. They believe in keeping the "truest form" of yoga. That we need to teach our students the way the poses were taught to us. And if I do not teach it that way, then we are not teaching "true yoga." I would not be surprised if we as Americans have in a way insulted the Indian culture calling how we practice yoga "yoga." I will say that was never my intent and I believe that was never the intent of other yoga instructors.

I also think the yoga is similar to religion (I DID NOT SAY YOGA IS A RELIGION). What I mean by this is that there are so many thoughts and perspective on what, how and why this or that is the best way to practice yoga. My personal opinion ... yoga can benefit anyone. The key is finding what style of yoga will benefit you, at this moment on your yoga journey.

We Americans do like to take old traditions and turn them into something "new and improved." And, in yoga, there's a reason for that: most Americans are not built for traditional yoga! Most Americans are nowhere close to being able to sit still unless it is on the sofa binge watching their favorite TV show let alone for two minutes on a yoga mat to meditate.

With all of that being said, there are amazing yoga instructors and now a slow-growing number of certified yoga therapists who have a much more training than an instructor with a 200-hour yoga teacher training certification. (Check out the **Learn More** page at the back of this book for more information.) I also believe that every yoga instructor has good intentions and are trying to help.

There is a shift to create better standards for training yoga instructors, calling for better overall certification standards, as well as more required continuing education. But, this shift will take time to design and implement.

Meanwhile, it's up to you to speak up, ask questions, and modify the poses as needed so your body can get as much of the full benefit of yoga to compliment you where you are on your journey.

That is why I am saying it is not all the yoga instructors fault. You need to research styles and types of yoga. Did you just jump behind the steering wheel of the car and start driving before you read some info on what the car could do? Or the rules of the road? If you heard a horn honked you pay attention. The same concept needs to be applied to your body.

You need to LISTEN to your body!

If an instructor is having you do something that you do not feel is right for you, then you need to listen to your horn if it's honking. I'll go over in more depth in Chapter 10 the dos and don'ts on how to keep yourself safe as you embark on your yoga journey. But before that, remember from the previous chapters the importance of continuing to move. I bet sometimes you feel like you want to move or workout. Yet you feel something is holding you back. There is something holding you back on an unconscious level. It's called kinesiophobia, which is the fear of movement.

This symptom of hypersensitivity from your fascia, your neuropathways, as well as the way you are moving all feed your kinesiophobia.

When this kinesiophobia kicks in, you unconsciously limit the amount of movement, range of motion and other behaviors and actions that you used to do on a daily basis. The unconscious behavior and thought process spill over to other physical activities you used to enjoy before your injury = or before your poor daily habits created your chronic issues.

Having a better understanding of why you think if you move your head a certain it may explode like a cartoon character, is going to supply you with a better understanding of the psychological aspects of your pain—the tricks our minds play on us. We'll do just that in the next chapter.

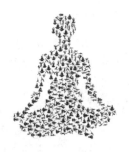

Fear is the path to the dark side.
Fear leads to anger.
Anger leads to hate.
Hate leads to suffering.

–Yoda

8

Catastrophizing and Kinesio what?

Fear is, I think, our biggest obstacle in just about anything we do. A fear of rejection, a fear of unacceptance by our family, peers and society. A fear of love. A fear of pain.

As I briefly mentioned in the last chapter, kinesiophobia is the fear of movement. This fear of movement can come from many different things, which I'll get into. A close cousin to kinesiophobia is catastrophizing (yes, that really is a word!)—a sort of projected fear. In this chapter, I'll give you simple ways to get past these sometimes debilitating fears.

To fear or not to fear. That is the question.

Let me start by saying, not all fear is bad. The Oxford dictionary defines fear as "an unpleasant emotion caused by the threat of danger, pain, or harm."

When you are out hiking in the woods and you hear a noise, a rustling in the bushes, or possible animal noises, you feel fear. It may be a cute deer or a grizzly bear depending on where you are. If you are walking down a dark alley at midnight, even if you are used to that area and feel perfectly comfortable during the day, you may feel fear at night for what could possibly be lurking in the shadows.

We feel fear when we think our safety has been compromised or will be compromised. That is normal. That is good. This fear is in anticipation of what may or may not happen and this healthy fear can protect us.

And then there's fear that's based on things our brain only *thinks* it's feeling or sensing, when there's no environmentally-based threat or danger.

Many times this fear has developed due to pain-related injuries, psychological distress or other various types of chronic pain.

Kinesiophobia is medically defined as an "irrational, weakening and devastating fear of movement and activity stemming from the belief of fragility and susceptibility to injury."[3] Many times this fear has developed due to pain-related injuries, psychological distress or other various types of chronic pain. Chronic pain can come for multiple different issues: post-traumatic stress disorder (PTSD), fibromyalgia, lower back pain, migraines, arthritis … and those are just a few.

Most likely your pain was brought on by a specific incident, event, or accident which put you in an acute injury stage. During this stage, in order for the healing process to be successful, you probably had to stay off your feet and take it easy for about four to eight weeks or longer. This is plenty of time to create bad habits *without even realizing you are doing it.*

Most people believe that in order for the injury to heal they need to not do any type of physical activity. This is not true. If possible, one of the best things you can do is to move as soon as possible. Of course, protecting and allowing the injury to heal, but if you have injured a lower body part, you could still use the arm crank machine to help with your upper body strength and aerobic health.

However, most people will not think of this option and are still frightful that even this upper body movement will cause their lower body injury harm.

In addition to not moving and limiting your movements consciously, you have more than likely been unconsciously over-compensating by holding your body differently trying to protect the injured part. This is perfectly natural and expected. Throughout this recovery process you have created stronger muscles, weaker muscles, tighter muscles and looser muscles a body full of imbalances in order to avoid doing more harm.

You have unconsciously limited your movements living in more of a one-dimensional world—overall not moving as much as you previously were—even though we are designed to live in a multi-dimensional world.

This fear of reinjuring yourself many times leads to catastrophizing, which is basically thinking and coming up with outcomes in your head, making things so much worse than they really are or will be.

The Sky is Falling!

Our brains can make the most illogical leaps. Here's how catastrophizing works in a nutshell:

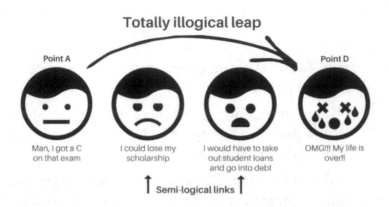

Totally illogical leap

Point A   Point D

Man, I got a C on that exam   I could lose my scholarship   I would have to take out student loans and go into debt   OMG!!! My life is over!!

↑ **Semi-logical links** ↑

Here's another example. Let's say it's now getting warmer, time to break out the shorts. Since you haven't seen your legs since last summer, you may not only be noticing the cellulite that old man winter has had us pack on the last couple of months, but now you notice a mole. As you start looking at it, you think it looks a little odd shaped. You go to the web to look up skin cancer moles. Wow. It looks really similar. Holy crap. You remember that your cousin three times removed had skin cancer. Holy shit. I've got skin cancer!!!!!!

Before you head to the dermatologist you've already diagnosed yourself that you have cancer and you're going to die.

Our brains do much the same thing with post-injury pain, even when the injury—the source of the pain—has healed.

In other words, most times you think your pain is a lot worse than it is. There are many reasons why you have started to catastrophize and many are very valid good reasons. Remember about the neuroplasticity in Chapter 4? Those pain pathways were traveled for a long period of time, which makes the memory of the incident vivid.

If you think back to your childhood, is there one special birthday you remember? Maybe a time when you got something you really wanted? Your memory is probably limited to the moment you opened that one special gift. In fact, do you even remember any of the other gifts?

How about an accident, maybe while you were riding a bike or a scooter—ever had a fall that you vividly remember because you sustained a really bad injury? Maybe it was a nasty cut that you still have a scar from. You remember that incident, right? What about all the other, more minor accidents you've had? I'm willing to bet your memory of those is vague, if you even remember them at all.

If you have children, maybe that memory of the bike accident comes back to you as you watch your child wobble down the sidewalk, trying to stay upright on two wheels. You warn your child over and over to "be careful." Each time they wobble—and, even worse, if they fall off—your body tenses up. Just like you would if you yourself were falling, you physically brace yourself on their behalf, tense up and may even feel pain. Your child may get up and be just fine, yet you experience a physical reaction to this fall because of a pain memory you had as a child. It's impossible to resist, because it's your body's natural reaction to your fear of them getting hurt based off of a memory, a neuropathway, when you experienced something similar.

I have a feeling that many of you associate your chronic pain with a certain activity or situation—an incident or accident that led to the initial injury and then the chronic medical issue. Maybe you were picking up your child when your back spasmed and you ended up in bed for two days, so now you hesitate before you sweep your child up in a hug. Or you were out for a run when you twisted your ankle and now whenever you pass that particular spot on your route, your ankle starts to hurt.

Your fear is limiting your actions and behaviors.

If you've ever been involved in a bad car accident, or even a fender bender, you know the feeling of panic that can set in when you see a car fast approaching behind you while you're slowing down. You think there is no way they're going to be able to stop in time. Your body starts to tense up, you grab the wheel or the passenger handle and brace for impact. You just can't help it. When the moment passes, you may even detect some pain in the area of your body that was injured in your previous accident. The pain memory of the previous accident is what causes you the pain, even though you have been healed for the last two years.

When you think back to that event, the body and the brain remember it. The body can feel the pain that was experienced before because the accident was learned and has created a memory—a neuropathway—in the brain. So, when the brain is noticing that this area, action or setting that is familiar, it will recall it and go on heightened alert to protect itself. It's a default.

So even though you were not hit this time, your brain was anticipating and catastrophizing from the previous experience. This may lead you to actually feeling that pain again where the injury took place. You may find your hands are shaking. Or you may feel anxious, nervous, or sad. Whatever other emotions you may have experienced with that moment. Mostly fear?

Why it is important for you to understand catastrophizing and kinesiophobia? So you can understand that your fear is holding you back from making yourself better. Your fear is limiting your actions and behaviors. This, many times, is the hardest concept to acknowledge. Once you admit to yourself that you have this fear, then you are able to address and figure out how to overcome this fear.

Research shows that individuals who have low risk and fairly routine knee arthroplasty (where they reconstruct or replace the joint) surgery, if the patient pain catastrophizes even a moderate amount, this is a strong indicator that the person will be disposed to developing chronic pain.[4] The higher level of pain catastrophizing before the surgery the more likely the patient would develop chronic pain after the surgery. The mindset before you even go into surgery seems to have an impact on if and how much chronic pain you may have after.

They are also finding that if individuals can get moving faster, this helps to limit the development of chronic pain.[5]

You are creating your future based on what you think might happen.

Remember that our brain is the hard drive of the body—constantly working, constantly sending out electrical impulses and signals throughout the body, moving us and controlling every action we make. Remember these brain cells (neurons) turn these electrical impulses into thoughts.

When you are sleeping, you dream. The brain is still working, still thinking, even when you are not awake. If you are stressed about something, many times you may have bad dreams that you can cause your stress.

What does this mean? The mind is a powerful thing. If you are thinking that you are going to be worse off, you many times will actually start believing it, which will cause you to start living it. You are creating your future based on what you think *might* happen.

Going back to neuropathways, or thought patterns, the more we travel a thought pattern the deeper that rut will become. Why do you think there are so many self-help books out there based on "positive thinking?" Because those thoughts influence our neurons, which influence our actions on a cellar level drastically! There is a lot of information out on the web that can provide you with some ways of coping and strategically getting through this catastrophizing and fear of movement. And please, it is OK to see some professional help in gaining control of this. Just because you see a professional does not mean you are crazy. It means you are being proactive it finding solutions in gaining back control of your life.

One simple example of not starting on this path to catastrophizing is try not to exaggerate.

Have you ever been around someone who is constantly thinking about the worst thing that can happen in a situation? They go on and on about how bad the traffic is going to be just running to the store, and how long they are going to have to wait in line. Simple things. Before they're ever out the door, the simple task of just running up the street or stopping off on their way home has turned into a negative, cumbersome task and just the thought of doing it has put them in a lousy mood. And you're left thinking, "Boy, dinner is going to be so pleasant tonight!" This negativity has a direct, negative impact on you.

Catastrophizing even this simple task has negatively swayed their mood, yet when they actually do the task, they may not experience a lot of traffic. Or stand in a long line at the store. They may be in and out in two minutes. *They are negatively impacting their present before they are even sure how their future may actually be.*

When it comes to pain catastrophizing, it is very similar in projecting pain into the future, yet it is related to a real event. Like I said previously, about the car wreck, in extreme cases there are some people who will not drive for long periods of time after a car accident because they are constantly afraid of something serious happening again.

Or if it's an action of going for a jog and the last time that happened their back seized up for days, they say they are never jogging again. The pain that they experienced was so excruciating, they never want to experience that again and therefore will never run again.

Those who pain catastrophize may say things like there is nothing that is ever going to fix their pain. And they are just going to have to suffer through it. Guess this is just how they are destined to live out the remainder of their life. Woe is me!

Being Present & Grounded Can Conquer the Fear

Some simple things you may want to try is really be present in what you are doing right now. If you are feeling good, or better than you were yesterday, acknowledge it. Be grateful that you are feeling better today and that you are experiencing a good day. This feel good feeling will trickle into other aspects of your day and many times makes other situations feel good as well. Remember that one positive neuron will have an impact on all of the other neurons.

Being more aware of how you are feeling at the moment will also help limit the negative thoughts of what may possibly happen to you later on. The future will be what it will be. And you do have control over it. Your actions and behaviors in this moment will have an impact on your future. So right now, enjoy this moment of feeling good.

There is the suggestion of good deep breaths. Do you remember your grandmother ever saying to you, "Just take a couple of good, deep breaths and everything will be fine"? Turns out, she was absolutely correct. Remember the vagus nerve I talked about in Chapter 5?

When you take those couple of good, deep breaths, your diaphragm communicates with your brain through that vagus nerve, stimulating the "parasympathetic" side of your nervous system. The parasympathetic side is in charge of relaxation, calmness, lowered blood pressure and heart rates, and digestion, among other functions. It's the "feel good" side of your nervous system.

Even if you enjoy gardening—and or wood working, knitting, cooking, baking, whatever you enjoy—doing these physical movements help you to reduce anxiety in that moment. Walking through the woods, or being in the garden, many people feel more grounded and connected to something greater than themselves. Nature seems to calm and relax people. If you think about it from the perspective that we all in a way are part of the world and we are all connected, this for some can be enough of an explanation. The warmth of the sun on our skin. The feel of the sand between our toes, the sound of ocean waved crashing on the shore. All of these can help people to feel relaxed and calm.

I mentioned in an earlier chapter, that yoga is about having a sense of being connected with the world, nature, the universe as well as other human beings in hopes of reaching self-realization and becoming our authentic selves. To bring harmony and balance to oneself mind, body, soul and with nature. Learning to be kinder to yourself so you are able to show kindness to others.

When practicing yoga, many of the poses give people a grounded feeling. This grounding is important to your catastrophizing and kinesiophobia because is provides you with security. When you feel safe you are able to pause and take a good look at the situation and what you are experiencing in that moment. Perspective on the situation and moment helps you to be more rational about the fear that you feel creeping in and helps to prevent catastrophizing.

When you feel that you have a good "footing" you have a sense of security.

Throughout a yoga class the instructor may make a comment about being grounded. It is common to hear instructors in the beginning of the class make references to imagine your feet are firmly rooted into the ground. Or visualize you are a strong oak tree and your toes becoming roots. For a newbie yogi like yourself you may not have a flipping clue what they're referring to. So here is a way of looking at it if you hear an instructor mention grounding.

Many of the Warrior poses have a sense of strength in the way you hold your arms, in the way that you position your legs. This feeling of strength provides a grounded, strong and energized feeling by the way they are holding their bodies. When you feel that you have a good "footing" you have a sense of security, not just physically but emotionally and mentally. If you are in down dog you literally have all "4's" on the ground. Two feet and two hands. These poses help people feel balanced, and creating a sense of calm, peace, and feeling safe in a world of crazy.

In savasana, corpse pose, final relaxation or nap time, many yoga practitioners favorite pose, your whole body is being supported by the ground. When relaxing you know that you are being supported and that you will not fall. You are safe.

If you have chronic pain you want to feel safe. You want to be in places situations and positions that will not cause you harm or remind you of being harmed. Totally understandable. If you continue to avoid becoming present in your life and keep running from possible things that may or may not harm you ... this is not good either. You can't run from your pain! You need to stand your ground and be proactive in combating your pain. Not running from it and be reactive.

You Can't Run from Pain

There is such a thing in the world of psychiatry called avoidance. People will avoid situations, other people, and places so they do not feel stress or anxiety and they do not have to acknowledge what is really bothering them. Dealing with the root cause of the pain is many times more uncomfortable than the actual physical pain itself. In trying to avoid possible triggers to their pain, they create other anxieties, and stressors running from the initial root cause of their pain. Possibly even turning towards other medications, drugs, alcohol or even mistaking their prescription pain medication.

Here's an example: I'll use a car wreck as the accident that lead to the initial pain. The individual who was injured in the wreck may not able to deal with the thought of getting into a car in fear of getting into another wreck. Understandable. So, they decide to take the bus, or Metro temporarily because they do have to get to work. Ok. This may be a great way for them to slowing get over their fear as well as limiting their footprint on the environment. Win win.

However, let's say that now this way of commuting is adding additional stress to the individual because they are having longer commute times, which lead to them missing their children's sporting events and other school activities.

Now their kids are disappointed because the parent didn't show. The other parent may be getting extremely frustrated that the injured parent is no longer pulling their weight with the children as well as around the house. Which leads to arguing among the parents, dealing with disappointed children who turn angry and resentful, and so on and so on.

To help with this avoidance, as well as the kinesiophobia, and catastrophizing guess what is extremely helpful? Yup. I've mentioned it before. Yoga.

Yoga is fundamentally about non-judgment of ourselves and others.

Yoga is a great way for people to be able to focus on themselves completely, even if it is for only ten to 50 minutes. As you move from pose to pose, you increase your dopamine levels as well as release tension throughout your muscles which help you to feel better. The breathing helps you to relax not just the body but helps you to get out of your head, even if only for a moment or two in the beginning.

When you feel calm throughout the body and the mind, this helps you be aware and able hear what the heart is trying to tell you. And no, I don't mean possible pounding of your heart that you feel in your head because you are out of shape. I'm referring to your emotions. Your feelings. To some feeling and emotions are the scariest thing of all. But if you keep pushing them off to the side, ignoring them and not addressing what you are feeling about the initial injury, accident, or the behaviors that you continue to act upon that contribute to your chronic pain, this emotional and mental discomfort exacerbates the physical discomfort.

Yoga is fundamentally about non-judgment of ourselves and others. (Funny how so many in the yoga world are extremely judgmental. But you'll find that in the religious world, too.) *Svadhyaya* is what is called a *Niyamas* in the yoga world. Things we should practice on a daily basis. It can be interpreted as self-study and non-judgment. Why this is important is we are quick to judge ourselves; negatively and positively. Too much negativity puts us on a slippery slope to a dark depressing pit. Too much ego and self-importance are looked as being arrogant, pompous, and being a prick, just to name a few. It's a hard balance to find.

Yoga creates a safe place for us to be with like-minded individuals who hopefully are there for the same reasons as you. To learn more about who they are providing a judge free space. This safe place helps you to let your guard down to lessen your anxiety and other stressors.

As you go through the poses, as I said, you feel a physical release which allows you to be more mindful of what you are emotionally feeling. Becoming aware of these feelings, positive or negative, and addressing these fears, or acknowledging these joys, is a catalyst in us becoming aware and acknowledging our bodies outside of the yoga room throughout our daily lives.

So, as you go through your daily life, and you start to catastrophize about your current situation or an upcoming one, or your kinesiophobia is kicking in, your yoga practice starts to provide you with friendly reminders and awareness about your present moment.

Ok. Great. So, I've given you the rationale as to why yoga works. Your doctor even may have recommended doing yoga and you may have numerous friends that swear by it. But you don't see how you'll fit into this yoga world. Your pain is different. Your pain is special. Sorry to bust your bubble ... but it's not.

Yoga can and will help your chronic pain tremendously!

I understand that you feel and think that your situation is different. And I am not trying to dismisses how you feel. Your feelings are yours and yours alone and they are real to you. I have no idea what you are feeling and experiencing. I am basing all of this off of the thousands of other patients and clients that I have worked with and helped. Whose stories are so similar to each other's sometimes I am in a parallel universe because I swear I just had this patient three months ago. (Oooh ... better yet, I'm in The Matrix. Or the movie *Groundhog Day*.) I'm just asking you to look at it from a different perspective.

I understand if you are resistant to the idea of walking into the boutique yoga studio on the corner having the instructor lead you into one crazy ass pose after another. You've seen some of those people in the studio, on TV and on the Internet. Just looking at some of those people in the poses make you hurt. (catastrophizing) Your lower back problems and pain are special. You hurt just from standing up straight. No way in hell you're headed to a yoga class that make your current pain even worse. How the hell is moving like that going to help? (kinesiophobia)

I don't blame you for feeling that way. Yoga can and will help your chronic pain tremendously! I have already explained several reasons why. The key is knowing how to keep yourself safe as you start on your yoga journey. Having the information and knowledge that I have given you about how your body is designed and supposed to move hopefully has given you better insight on simple things that could potentially aggravating your current chronic pain condition. If nothing else, I hope I've at least provided you with some information to help you become more self-aware.

This self-awareness may provide you insight as to why you have been self-sabotaging your health and your happiness. I am not saying that you are doing it on purpose. I honestly do not believe anyone would do that to themselves on purpose.

If no one has told you, I will tell you. You *do* deserve to be happy and healthy. **You are worthy of being happy and healthy!** I do care about your happiness. Why? If I believe in the yoga philosophy that nature, the universe, and everyone on this Earth is connected and intertwined, your happiness impacts those of others. In the next chapter, I'm going to tackle an often uncomfortable topic, with (I hope) a lot of love and of course, a bit of humor!

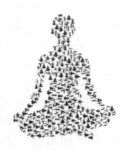

Who in the world am I?
Ah, that's the great puzzle.
–Lewis Carroll, Alice in Wonderland

9

You Deserve to Be Healthy

I want to take a moment to address the obesity epidemic. And before you jump my shit and say I just called you fat, keep reading. I'm going to be getting onto anyone who is out of balance and living an extreme.

Remember I just said in the previous chapter, I *do* care, and you are worthy of being happy and healthy. So, I am asking you to please be open minded to this topic.

I want you to be honest with yourself. You *need* to be honest with yourself if you want to have a chance at diminishing your chronic pain and or getting a hold of it and living the life you desire. I am going to ask you questions. You may know what the answers are right away. You may not know the answers a week from now or a year from now. Or if ever. That is okay. You don't have to have all the answers. In fact, my definition of wisdom is ... I do not have all the answers.

As I ask these questions, feel free to speak it out loud into the book. (I promise I won't tell anyone.) When you speak out loud this allows you to hear what you said. For whatever reason when you think something it doesn't sound so bad. You know the context in how you are thinking it. But then you say it out loud there are times you can't believe that actually sounded good in your head.

Example, I feel I am genetically disposed to having a flat ass. I have been in pursuit of making my flat ass more muscular and fuller for years. The other day a woman walked by and I thought, "I totally want her ass." If I had said this out loud it may not have come across the way I was thinking it to someone hearing me say it out loud nearby.

When you say your answers out loud, they may have a different effect on you than when you are just thinking them. Research shows that speaking out loud helps us to organize our thoughts. Many times we are able to visualize what we want, but articulating these wants and thoughts is another ball game. If you are afraid of being honest with yourself, ask why. What are you afraid of finding out? (There is that damn word fear again.) I want to be very clear that I am addressing these topics because I care. I am coming from a place of compassion and I am coming from a place of non-judgment. More than likely, you are your own worst critic.

There's No Weigh Around This

A third of the adult U.S. population has some type of lower back pain. Once again, I know. A shocker. So, how do you help to alleviate your lower back pain? One, start paying attention to what you are eating, how much water you are drinking and how active you are. One of the first and best things you can do for yourself is to lose some weight. I am saying this to you because you more than likely you are drastically fudging and just plain lying to yourself that you do not have any weight to lose. You like who you are, curves and all. "I'm not fat. A size 12 is not fat or overweight. I am in my ideal body weight." More than likely you are not.

Did you know that, according to the Centers for Disease Control, as of November 2, 2012, the average height for a female adult over the age of 20 was 63.8 inches (5ft 3 inches), 166.2 pounds with a waist circumference of 37.5 inches? If you plug those numbers into a generic BMI calculator (body mass index), which you can find pretty much anywhere online, that is 29.4 BMI. The number 29.4 falls into the category of overweight by CDC calculations, and a BMI of 30.0 is considered obese. So, the "average" female adult is just 0.6 points away from being considered obese!

More than two-thirds (68.8 percent) of adults are considered to be overweight or obese. And more than one-third of adults (35.7 percent) are considered to be obese. More than 1 in 20 people are considered to be extremely obese. And then you wonder why your back hurts, or you get headaches.

Intentions are not actions.

Reality check. Ask yourself, do you fit into one of these categories? If the answer is yes, then you can start being proactive in making changes to help improve your body and mind. Do you go to a yoga class which the doctor said would be good for you? Do you make the changes that you need to with your nutrition, your sleep and activity? I'm taking a wild guess and saying you think you are taking the right step, but you are probably making a half-ass attempt at it, or at least have the best intentions. Intentions are not actions.

I'm not saying this to be mean. I am saying this because I care. I want you to live a happy, healthy, full, active life. This life and world is amazing and watching it from the couch on the TV or your laptop does NOT count as actually living it.

Not only are you more than likely lying to yourself about your weight, but also lying to yourself that you enjoy and are happy watching life pass you by and play out on some reality show like "The Real Cowboys of the West" or "The Fantastic World of the Rich and Crazy."

And then in between your binge watching to get caught up what Tina did when her custom pink cowgirl boots came in the wrong shade of pink, the marketing companies are lying to you telling you that all of your problems can be fixed by some new and improved diet, or drug, or exercise. And in only seven days! It's a lie that obtaining your goals and all the things you want out of life can and will be effortless.

But that's what companies want you to believe. Just take a pill, eat this, drink this kind of water, or use this new exercise equipment. All you need to do is hook your abs up to some electric device and, in no time flat—*snap!*—you'll have a six pack.

It's so easy to buy into the easy, quick fix. These quick fixes tell us it won't take a lot of time, it will be easy, effortless and will solve all of your problems so you can go live with your prince charming and live happily ever after.

They are all enablers. Your family, your friends the commercials and TV shows and society who are all telling you what you want to hear. And that is why you are buying.

I'm not going to be an enabler (someone who helps the person stay where they are).

I am not going to lie to you and tell you what you want to hear because you are already getting that from plenty of other sources. I want you to succeed and sustain your success so I'll be honest with you.

So yes. You are probably overweight if not in the obese category. If so, yes, the weight more than likely is contributing to some of your chronic pain. Yes, the weight is going to take some time to come off. Yes, it will be hard. Yes, you do have to do more than just work out or eat right. Yes, you will stay in your current state unless you start making good conscious choices on a regular basis. Yes, you are the only one that can make these changes. And yes, every time you have a reason why you are not able to make these changes ... it's just an excuse.

The good news is that you can make all of these changes! Doing yoga will help alleviate some of your discomfort while you are doing other physical activities and making other lifestyle changes to reduce your weight as well as bring awareness and helping you become more mindful in your choices while on your new healthy happy path.

Finding Your Authentic Self

I care if you are healthy. I care you are happy. This world if a pretty fucking amazing place. How you live your life and the choices you make have no direct impact on my life at this moment. But they do have a direct impact on your life and those of your friends and your family. So the reason I care ...

it's the yogi in me. Even though I just said that your choices do not directly impact my life at this moment, does not mean that your life does not impact mine at some point, or that you are not impacting someone else's at this moment.

Remember early on in the book I explained that yoga is about bringing the mind, body and spirit of a person into harmony and balance. How every individual is intertwined in some way with other humans, the earth, nature and the universe and beyond. Everyone has their difference of options as to what and how they believe or even if they believe this at all. That is what is so great about free will.

I believe in energy. Everything is energy. Even inanimate objects have some type of energy that the human eye is not able to see. With that being said, I believe that happiness is energy. If you are happy and healthy, you bring happiness into others' lives that you encounter throughout your day. The saying, "I like their vibe. I like their energy" is because living creatures pick up on others' energy.

OK, OK ... stay with me a bit longer. I'm going somewhere with this hippie dippy crap.

Understanding your authentic self helps you to gain a better understanding of your fears.

I personally feel that yoga is a tool that helps an individual become their authentic self. We all struggle in this world to feel loved and to feel that we belong. And we tend to change our behaviors and thoughts when needed so we will be accepted and loved. The problem comes into play when we stop being our authentic selves for extended periods of time.

When we are younger, we are still trying to figure out who we are and where we belong. That's common and natural. As we grow into our authentic selves we will change our behaviors and thoughts as we gain better understanding of who we are.

Having a better understanding of who we are, being honest with ourselves is extremely challenging. This better understanding of who you are provides insight as to why you react, respond, and continue the behaviors you do on a daily basis. Healthy or unhealthy. Understanding your authentic self helps you to gain a better understanding of your fears. And many times, when you are finally able to have a better understanding of your fears and accept your authentic self, this leads you to have more compassion for those around you.

The first step in gaining better understanding of yourself is to ask the questions. Why do you feel this way? Asking these questions can be scary. Many times we don't want to ask ourselves this question because we are afraid of the answer. (There's that damn fear thing again.) If you do not know the answer, ask and listen to what others are afraid of. This may help spark an ah-ha moment. A brief moment of clarity. When you gain deeper clarity of your fears, you are then able to figure out a strategy to help you overcome these fears.

However, many times we know the answers, but are unsure of how to change these fears. Or we have tried several times before and we were hurt or failed. So, we think if we keep ignoring them, they will magically disappear on their own. This avoidance of acknowledging these fears many times leads to our poor choices, and our chronic pain. We use other things (food, drugs, alcohol, shopping, etc.) to try to occupy ourselves so we are able to avoid confronting our fears. You need to address these fears. And if the mind and the heart are not going to acknowledge them, the body will.

When we start having health issues, many times it is because we are not attending to or acknowledging one or more of our health components. We may be exercising, eating right, yet our sleep is off because you keep having crazy ass dreams that a chipmunk (you saw a cute one in the park the other day) on a cheetah (a.k.a. your car that needs to have $500 worth of maintenance done) coming after you with a cattle prod (symbolizing your looming work deadline).

I don't know about you, but dreams like this are common for me. And when I acknowledge the stress, it leads me to my fear. And when I have a better understanding about my fear, I am then able to come up with a strategy to kick its ass.

Yoga is about compassion and kindness. In order to achieve overall health, it is learning how to be kind to yourself. It is learning to extend compassion to yourself. Many of us find it easy to extend compassion and kindness to others, yet we feel that we are not worthy of giving it to ourselves. Why?

Being healthy is more than just the physical superficial exterior appearance.

When we start to slowly extend compassion and kindness to ourselves, our authentic self starts to feel safe enough to come out of hiding. (You notice I just said the opposite of fear? I said safe.) When we feel and realize that the only one that is going to make us happy, to give us kindness, compassion and that we are worthy of being healthy and happy, your choices and behaviors start to emulate this understanding.

The Amazing Machine

Being healthy is more than just the physical superficial exterior appearance. The exterior appearance can show a healthy happy individual. And they may be. But it can be very deceiving about someone's health as well.

Don't get me wrong, someone who is in shape, eats well, gets good sleep, is hydrated and looks sexy as hell is very healthy. They almost seem to glow. I think that those that seem to glow, their physical health is good as well as their mental and emotional. I believe that health comes from the inside and radiates out.

There are sexy ass people who eat right and exercise yet still have high cholesterol, blood pressure and are at higher risk of a stroke or heart attack. They may have to take a pill anyways. Genetics. I have many friends of mine who carry extra weight and they can totally kick my ass in a run. If I trained harder I would be able to run better. I may still never be a better runner than they are, but I could be more proactive in my training. So, with that in mind, ask yourself have you been as proactive as you can, and doing everything that is in your control to help your body, mind and spirit be healthy? Or have you been defaulting and using the excuse of genetics as a scapegoat?

I want you to turn your thoughts to your internal health. What you are not able to see with your eyes. Take a moment and pause and ask yourself if the extra weight that you may be carrying could be causing your chronic pain? If you were to look at your heart, joints, or brain do you think they would look healthy? Would they be pink and reddish tints of color due to increased blood flow, nutrients and oxygen? What would your emotional and mental health internal health look like?

When I speak of health, I am talking about the mind, body, heart and soul. It is not only about eating the right things but it is exercising, getting proper sleep and hydration. It is about emotional and mental wellbeing and healthy positive relationships with others in your life. These all need to be balanced. These are called *chakras* in the yoga world.

You can try to separate them, ignore them and pay attention to some more than others. Many of us do this without realizing it. We tend to pay attention more to the ones that don't require as much work. They don't require as much work because we find them fun and enjoy doing them. Since we keep up with things we enjoy, they get more attention than the others and are not as challenging when we pay attention.

Your body is an amazing machine. Let's say this machine looks like a Ferrari. (Or whatever car you want it to be.) And this car has been cared for throughout the years. The body is sleek, lean and easy on the eyes. The engine roars and can get you from point A to point B in a heartbeat all while enjoying a comfortable smooth ride. Everyone wants to drive a Ferrari.

But what happens when you don't wash or wax the body of the car? What if this Ferrari's engine (the brain) has not had the oil changed since it was purchased, and what if the interior seats (the heart) have not been cared for and are cracking because that ice cream spill was never wiped off? And if you put diesel fuel in an unleaded car, it's no longer a comfortable ride as the car is jerking as it goes down the road because you fueled it with something it is not designed to utilize to run smoothly. You would not want nor be able to drive that car.

I like the car analogy, so let's break it down.

The body of the car = the human body:

If you want to keep the classic car's paint shining you need to wash it, cover it in harsh weather conditions and buff it. If you enjoy physical exercise more than likely the human body is going to be easier to maintain so working out is not as challenging the more you do it. I bet the human body gets buffed more often as well. (Let your mind take you somewhere with that. Mine did).

The interior of the car = the human heart:

Emotional health is important for those you are in relationships with and more importantly with YOURSELF. It takes time and effort to understand how others feel and even more so how and why you feel the way you do about situations and things. Having a better understanding of your emotions and others helps provide an easier ride. Cleaning the interior of the car and conditioning the leather interior seats this will provide better comfort to those that you invite to accompany you on this ride called life.

The engine = the human brain:

In order to keep the mind sharp and alert, giving it things like education, brain puzzle exercises, and physical exercise (I know you probably didn't want to hear that word again) is like changing the oil regularly and making sure the spark plugs are firing by cleaning them so they do not get covered with corrosion.

Fuel for the car = nutrition for the body:

Everyone knows that you do not put diesel fuel in an unleaded car. If you do, the engine will not run and you'll end up on the side of the road stranded waiting for a tow truck. So why do we expect our bodies to run smoothly and efficiently when we fuel it with diesel (high fructose corn syrup, sugar, etc.)?

Finding the Balance

I know those who fall into the category of being overweight, obese, underweight, or too skinny have tried multiple times to lose the extra weight or gain extra weight. Genetics can play a role in how your body absorbs and utilizes food. Genetics also play a role in how your body is predisposed to looking, i.e. hourglass, pear, etc. The type of exercises that people are able to do, and how their body uses and burns the fat, medical conditions as well as how you grew up and what you were exposed to are all contributing factors when it comes to overall health.

Not everyone's body is going to like the low carbs diets. Not everyone's body will respond well to eliminating meat from their diet. Not everyone's body is going to like being dairy free. Or gluten free. There are healthy foods that people eat knowing they are eating healthy foods, yet they are not able to lose the weight or gain the weight because they are actually allergic to them. This allergy will inflame the brain and the body possibly leading to chronic pain. And I am not just taking about dairy and gluten. I'm talking about corn. Something that does not get a lot of press. And if you have looked into or heard how they genetically modify our food these days, it is a bit disturbing. And too much to get into now.

An extreme is not balanced.

What many of these do have in common ... they are extremes. An extreme is not balanced. And when the body is not balanced, it gets stressed. And the funny thing is, many people will use extremes as a way to control and avoid their fears.

Stress—physical, mental and emotional—is a huge contributing factor in whether a person is able to lose the weight or not. When you are stressed your body will go into survival mode. For some that means their bodies will hold onto fat. They will stress eat. For others, they lose their appetite and do not eat.

There is such a thing as skinny fat. There are those that eat, but exercise too much trying to burn off the calories they ate. Or they are really good about their diet to stay skinny, but they do not exercise. Your body needs exercise. There are extremes in exercising as well. Those who exercise for hours a day so they can eat whatever they want. Or those who do repeated exercises to the point of causing themselves physical damage in the name of bigger biceps. Anorexia, bulimia, as well as extreme diets that limit specific foods. I believe all start out with good intentions but when taken to extremes they create multiple health concerns. The balance is gone.

Overweight people can have chronic pain in their joints and muscles due to carrying around extra weight the body is not designed to carry. Skinny people experience chronic pain because the body's tissues are not being nourished due to improper nutrition, and/or they're not exercising causing poor muscular strength in supporting their spine and other joints. Those who excessively exercise have chronic pain because they do not allow their bodies enough recovery time to heal from the previous constant repeated pounding they inflict on their bones and muscles.

The obesity epidemic is real. People are dying from being too overweight and fat. People are dying from anorexia from being skinny fat. People are dying from straining their internal organs by taking too much of some things and not enough of others.

There needs to be balance. Yoga provides us balance. Physically, mentally, and emotionally.

I want you to be honest with yourself about if you fit into one of these categories. If you do, ask yourself if you know why? I know that can be an extremely complex question. Being overweight, or too skinny, or following extreme diets or extreme exercising typically have had many layers added on throughout the years.

I will say this. I once again want to make it very clear that I am NOT a licensed phycologist, nutritionist, medical provider of any kind. And I am also NOT promising that I am going to "cure" your chronic pain or "fix" you. So when I ask this question, just take it for what it is. A question.

Do these extremes give you control? Or do these extremes make you feel out of control? Or both? Do you like how these extremes make you feel? If not, what do you NOT like about these feelings?

This will not be easy. You will have set backs. You will have good days and bad days. That is life. That is living.

Would you like to gain control of your pain? Would you like to gain a better understanding of yourself so you are able to understand your fears about your pain? Do you cling to this pain and identify with it in some way?

Do you feel you deserve this pain? Do you feel you are worthy of being healthy and happy?

Do your authentic self a favor and really try to answer these questions. Write them down. Ponder them. You don't need an answer right now. Just start conquering your fears by being brave enough to ask the questions.

If you have to, think to yourself, "I am worthy of health and happiness."

And then say it out loud.

I've said it before and I will say it again, this will not be easy. You will have set backs. You will have good days and bad days. That is life. That is living.

A friend of mine, Mike Waldron, is the Executive Director of the nonprofit 23rd Veteran. He's paying it forward and doing some pretty fantastic things for veterans who are suffering from PTSD. He offers a resiliency training program with positive psychology. There are many things offered in the program, yoga and meditation being one of them. (And yoga is a great tool to help recondition yourself with positivity.)

I think the program is badass. I think their slogan is even more badass:

"Happiness is not an entitlement, you have to earn that shit."

Show yourself some kindness in doing something healthy like going for a walk or eating an apple. Tell yourself that you are allowed and deserve to be happy and healthy.

If you or anyone else has never said it to you before, I will tell you:

You Are Worthy of Being Healthy and Happy!

I will believe in you until you start to believe it.

Start being honest with yourself so your authentic self can start to come out of hiding.

And as you start to slowly venture out of hiding into the yoga world, you're in luck as I've learned some tricks and tips in keeping you safe as you embark on this journey of health in how to control or in learning how to manage your chronic pain.

In the next chapter I provide you with those tricks and tips in keeping you safe as you start earning your happiness.

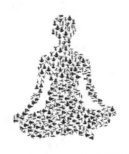

Yoga does not just change
the way we see things,
it transforms
the person who sees.

–B.K.S. Iyengar

10

The Dos and Don'ts of Yoga

The first do of practicing yoga: Just do it!!! If you only have time for a couple of sun salutations, or doing some spinal twists at your desk, then do that. If you only have five minutes in every hour, then do some yoga. Or if you want to call them stretches I don't care. But once again, yoga has been around long before the word "stretches" probably existed in our western society.

I don't care what you call it, as long as you're doing it and it works for you and your issues.

This chapter is where everything you've learned about your magnificent brain and body comes into play with your yoga practice.

Motion is Lotion

Throughout this book I've laid out some very specific physical reasons why movement in general and yoga in particular can help your chronic pain. It all comes down to this: motion is lotion.

That's not just a cute saying; the "lotion" is called synovial fluid. Synovial fluid is a viscous fluid that is found in the cavities of synovial joints. A synovial joint is one of the most common and most movable types of joint in the body, like knees and elbows. And the synovial fluid is what helps to prevent friction between the cartilage in synovial joints during movement.

Less synovial fluid means the potential of increased painful movement. Did you know that if you are lacking synovial joint fluid that one of the best ways in increase this is to do exercise?

The synovial fluid is important because it helps to keep the joints lubricated and provides cushioning. Cartilage does not have its own blood supply and needs to rely on carriers that transport and provide nutrients and hydration to joints of the body.

So, when you move—like doing yoga—you help to nourish the cartilage that helps to buffer the joints. When you increase blood flow, nutrients and oxygen to your body, whether it is cartilage, muscles, ligaments, or tendons, you are able to increase your recovery/healing time. When the body gets the food that it needs, then it can heal, grow and get healthier. Not to mention, physical exercise like yoga helps to make the muscles stronger providing better support to the skeletal system.

Remember the fascia from Chapter 6? How it helps to transport fluids throughout the body to keep it hydrated as well as to the discs between your vertebra and other joints?

Movement improves the range of motion in our joints and helps our fascia to stay hydrated.

Friendly reminder about hydration and the discs between your vertebrae being like a kitchen sponge: I previously mentioned to drink half your body weight in ounces a day in water. Remember, that's *on top of and in addition* to the 1 to 1 ratio for caffeine or alcohol (i.e., if you have 10 oz. of coffee, you need an additional 10 oz. of water). I know it's a lot of water, by if it could prevent a migraine wouldn't you rather have to pee a lot?

Now that you know that motion is lotion, are you likely to move and do yoga? It is low impact, a great way to increase muscular strength and increase flexibility while keeping your body and its tissues healthy. When you have a better understanding why yoga helps, you're (hopefully) more likely to keep moving.

The 5 Rules of Yoga

If you take away nothing else from this book, please remember these underlying rules of yoga. (At least they're my rules.) These are going to keep you safe, get you the results that you want, and limit the possibly for more potential injury. (If you're worried about that.)

Rule No. 1:

There is no gain in pushing through the pain!

A sharp, stabbing, radiating, shooting pain is NOT normal. If you are experiencing any of these I would highly encourage and recommend that you ease off. I'm not asking you to stop moving though. Think of it this way. My mentor, an absolute brilliant, amazing physical therapist and just an overall great guy and fantastic human being, Jeff Frankart, had the best way of explaining this feeling.

Pretty much everyone drives a car. And everyone has seen the tachometer on the dashboard. This tachometer lets you know how many RPMs (revolutions per minute) or how fast the engine is turning. There is a red line on this gauge that tells you if you do not shift gears or do not let off the gas and keep pushing through this red line, you'll blow your engine. So you downshift or just let off the gas as the needle gets to the red line. You don't slam on the brakes. If you do you could send yourself into a tailspin right off the road.

Another example is if you're on ice and you start sliding, slamming on your brakes would be a bad thing to do. Once again, you just let off the gas or downshift.

It's the same thing with your movement. This sharp, stabbing, shooting radiating pain, is your red line. If you keep pushing through your redline, you'll blow your engine. (Not necessarily your heart or brain, but that body part where you are feeling that pain.) Just ease off. Don't stop moving, but do modify the movement or position, and decrease your intensity or your weight.

Remember, movement helps to desensitize you. So, if you find as you are moving you think you are in pain, ease off, ask yourself is it sharp, stabbing, shooting or radiating? If it takes you longer than three seconds to figure out if you are in pain, you're more than likely not. If it is none of those, more than likely you are just uncomfortable. And life is uncomfortable.

Rule No. 2:

Always try to create distance and space between your vertebrae.

Why is this so important? Because we are trying to undo what gravity and the weight of our bodies do to us on a daily basis. That is a price we pay for walking upright. If you have disc or nerve issues, which many of you have, creating space between the vertebrae is going to help alleviate pressure off of those discs and possibly nerves if that is one of your issues. You will hear many times to "sequence the spine" or "roll the spine up one vertebra at a time" as I mentioned previously. While we do need to move our spines in multiple directions, it is designed to do that for a reason, we limit ourselves on a daily basis and when we do start moving our spines need to be eased into it. Flare ups may occur because we end up pinching the discs or nerves by hanging out in a rounded position. Pivot from your hips and try to be mindful of keeping space between your vertebrae and in a neutral alignment.

Rule No. 3:

Always have an over-exaggerated posture.

This and Rule No. 2 go hand in hand. If you try to imagine creating space between your vertebrae, observe what your body does. Bet you stand up straighter. Fun fact: You want to look like you lost five pounds instantly? Stand up straight. Yes, even though you do want to move and round your spine, you will not be able to maintain this over-exaggerated posture throughout an entire yoga class. But if you are mindful of trying to create this over-exaggerated posture throughout your yoga practice as it will keep you safe in most of the yoga poses, and it will limit the potential of overloading your facet joints and aggravating your back. It will also help to get you a deeper stretch.

When you hinge at your hips where you are supposed to while keeping an over-exaggerated posture, it is hard to round your back almost forcing you to pivot from your hips. Your back will thank you later. This over-exaggerated posture will also help to keep you in more of your "true form" which will increase the stretch, activate the muscles and keep you safer in the pose. Many times yoga instructors instruct the students roll or sequence the spine up from a forward fold. (Have you noticed I mentioned this a lot throughout the book?) Or to keep their legs straight, when they go into forward fold. Not good for the spine!

I should make this another one of my underlining rules, but never lock out your knees, especially on a forward fold. You overload your facet joints by 10x the amount of load they are designed to handle and possibly pinch nerves and discs which can lead to a flare up. I mentioned previously about how it is not wise to hang out with a rounded spine or posture for long periods of time. I know it's hard to resist. It probably feels good at the moment with those feel-good endorphins kicking in because the muscle is able to relax. But I wouldn't recommend it. This may feel good in the moment (just like not wearing a condom) but the complications that come after can be alarming.

Rule No. 4:

DO NOT EVER apply pressure to the top of your head!

I'm going to get a lot of crap from the yoga community for saying this, I'm sure. And I'm okay with that. If it means keeping you safe and limiting potential flare ups for you, I'll take the heat. Doing a head stand is one of the most thought-of yoga poses. Almost the Holy Grail of yoga poses.

However, here's my rationale and reasoning behind this rule. The conversation with other instructors goes a little like this: *"But if you teach them to do the head stand correctly only ten percent of their body weight should be applied to their head. And if they do it correctly they should be using their core, shoulders and arms to hold them upright. And if you don't have them do headstands then they are missing out on all of the benefits from an inversion."*

OMG!!! First off, that's a lot of ifs. Second, I have seen instructors teach people how to use their head as a pedestal to get themselves up into a wheel (*chakrasana* or full bridge)—which is basically a 180 degree backbend. The angle at which you're applying pressure to the cervical spine is very dangerous. The neck is not designed to take that amount of pressure at that angle. And if your arms and shoulders are that weak and lack the flexibility, you are not ready to go up into a full bridge. My personal opinion.

Some yoga instructors might protest my advice, arguing for the benefits of inversion, like improved circulation and venous return (letting gravity help your veins do their job). Guess what? A down dog is an inversion. But think of this logic, Sam logic ... if the average human head weights eight to 11 pounds, and only ten percent of the body weight should be on the head, who in that yoga class weights 80 to 110 pounds, give or take and doing it correctly?

If you have been practicing yoga, I bet you have been in a yoga class where the instructor says, "If it is in your practice feel free to do a headstand." People start to do head stands and if you have peeked and looked around for wall space because you're afraid you'll take out your neighbor, did you see people using their heads as pedestals to balance shaking because they are lacking strength in their abs, shoulders and arms? If you haven't, I bet you will. Or this may have even happened to you. You may have even done it because the "Keeping up with the Jones" mentality kicked in (aka the ego). Think of all that weight and pressure being applied to the cervical spine. And then they wonder why they get headaches.

If you are prone to headaches and migraines I would highly encourage and recommend that you DO NOT apply pressure to the top of your head. And if you do ... I told you so.

Rule No. 5:

Learn to be comfortably uncomfortable.

There *is* such a place as being comfortable with discomfort, and this is the place where you want to be. Growth comes from being uncomfortable. Discomfort helps you learn to connect to your body, mind and spirit as to why you feel the discomfort. (And possibly introduce you to muscles that you never knew you had.) This discomfort is when you can really be aware of what exactly is creating it.

Once again, when you are able to figure out where your discomfort is stemming from (fear, avoidance, emotional pain, self-doubt, laziness), acknowledging the discomfort is the first step in gaining back control of your pain. Then once you are able to acknowledge the discomfort sometimes you need or have to stay uncomfortable for a while. This is when your breath can give you power. In yoga breath is called *pranayama*. It translates to *life force*. I think it's very suiting. If you're not breathing, more than likely you're dead or will be soon. It still blows my mind when I think that there is just no way that I can hold the pose or stretch any longer, taking a deep breath can completely relax your body. The breath helps to still the mind and the body so you are able to be in the moment and not feel the need to run from it.

(Note: If you're having trouble keeping up with the breath-to-movement patterns throughout the class, just keep breathing. Don't hold your breath and pass out. Probably should be another Rule.)

Learning how to deal with being uncomfortable is going to help you in your everyday life. Why? Being uncomfortable many times stems from fear. This fear leads to stress. When your stress levels kick into high gear with your career, kids, friends, just life in general, learning how to stay calm in the storm is the key to staying sane and functioning in the moment.

The Dos of Yoga

DO #1: Question what the instructor is telling you.

I know this will piss off some yoga instructors that want you to be quiet, listen to your body and your inner voice. Many practice yoga to find the calm and the peace. While understand this and agree, for those that are dealing with chronic pain, I have found that many need to have a better understanding of how they can be calm when their back is on fire. Out of respect, if you are able to speak with the instructor before the class, all the better. Ask them if it's okay to ask questions that directly pertain to the pose and why should do it this way or that throughout their class. If you wait until after the class is over to ask, it could be too late. If they say sure, and during the class an answer they give you doesn't sit right with you, then do a modification and remember one of my rules. Then, when you get a chance, do your own research and seek another yoga instructor.

Many of these yoga instructors have been taught in more traditional styles of yoga practices. The chances are good that a few people in your yoga class have some kind of medical issue. (The Centers for Disease Control states that about half of adults have at least one chronic health condition such as cancer, obesity, arthritis, etc.). With many overweight, deconditioned and injured individuals that are just getting out of acute injury rehab or have other chronic diseases, the instructors, more often than not, may not be able to give the best advice on modifications for you and your particular issues. Especially if they only have a 200-hour certification. If they want you to do a pose a specific way, ask them why. Chances are, other students in the class have the same question, or did at one time, and are afraid to speak up. If the instructor gets upset and tells you to do it because they said so, or you need to be quiet because you're interrupting students' zen, well, I wouldn't go back. But that's just me.

Albert Einstein was such a wise man. He said, "Question everything." And another personal favorite, "Logic will get you from A to B. Imagination will take you everywhere."

Imagination helps us to think outside our boxes. To find what we are able to do and what is best for us. It's all about perspective.

DO #2: Always ALWAYS listen to your body.

A sharp, stabbing, shooting, or radiating pain is **not normal**. This is your body's way of telling you that something is not right and you should probably ease off (see Rule No. 1 above). You want to be comfortably uncomfortable. (Rule No. 5). Yoga is great for showing us in a short amount of time what our bodies really can and should not do. There is no way to ignore it when you are trying to do a pigeon pose. It will let you know what is going on if you listen to it.

DO #3: Do as your body is requesting!!

(And if your body is requesting that you don't move, refer to DON'T #4.) We can listen to our bodies all day long, but when we do not do what it is asking, like move from behind our desks and stretch about every half hour, and you end up on the floor at night because your back is spasming, are you really that surprised? The human body is an amazing, wise machine. If we listen to it, and then do as it is requesting, it will be a lot happier with us.

But when we don't, it will talk back to us and let us know how ticked off it is. Whether that is by back spasms, or our stomachs get upset, or we get headaches and migraines. These are many times indicators that we are not giving our body want it needs.

We might think we're smarter than our bodies because we Googled our symptoms or are following the newest and latest food and exercise fad. The body is talking to us all day. Yet we ignore it. What happens when your toddler gets ignored? They keep pulling on your shirt or dress, and then finally start screaming when they are tired of being ignored. Your body will do the same thing.

DO #4: Remember that your body is amazing.

Why do I keep saying that? Because every seven to ten years, every cell in your body is new. How cool is that? It's like a fresh start. How you choose to treat those new cells can not only impact your present but also your future.

And **DO** remember that our thoughts impact the function of our cells. Think about it this way. Our mind controls every action of our bodies. It's the hard drive. It controls how we move, when we move, what we eat, and how we eat. That includes our thoughts. Positive thoughts can strengthen your immune system, and negative thoughts can make us sick.

DO #5: When in doubt, use your legs.

Why do I say this? Because your leg muscles are one of the largest and strongest groups of muscles in your body. Many of those that have back pain are in a habit of moving throughout their daily lives with their backs in poor positions. Their backs are typically deconditioned and weak. They forget that their legs are so strong and to use their legs to work for them, not against them.

What I mean is that in many yoga *asanas*, if someone is feeling it in their back, they are typically using their backs, not their legs or abdominals. In many yoga poses the instructor will cue you to lift up the body, like in a bridge pose and say try not to use the legs. While I understand why they say this, for those that have chronic back pain, I recommend that you do use your legs to assist you while you gain strength in your back. And really use your legs and glutes especially if you are lifting your leg into a pose like Warrior III. If you are not activating your glutes, quadriceps and hamstrings and just letting your leg hang behind you, you are now adding extra resistance and pull to your lower back. This will aggravate the back. This is why it's important to modify and do what you are capable of—not pushing yourself into the next pose just to say you can do it.

DO #6: Do remember to *mula bandha*.

That's Sanskrit for "suck it in" like one of your top five just walked into the room. It's actually more of a deep pelvic root lock. It is called imprinting if you have ever done Pilates. Why is this important? Your abdominal muscles are connected to your hips/pelvis and your pelvis is the middle ground of your body. If you contract those muscles this will aid in a slight tilt of your pelvis positioning it under your rib cage where they it is biomechanically designed to go. Remember in the Kinetic Chain chapter how your body fights over your pelvis? If your leg muscles are tight, they will be trying to pull the pelvis towards them putting more strain on the lower back.

You may have heard in a fitness classes to "tuck your pelvis under." You do not want to do a huge posterior pelvic tilt forward as this will move the hips too far forward in the opposite direction creating additional strain or other discomfort in your lower back. It's a balance.

I'd like you to try something for me. Put your hands on your hips. Suck in your gut and be mindful of what happens to your shoulders. What did you feel? Did you feel yourself stand up straighter? The kinetic chain, baby.

DO #7: Do set yourself a goal.

I don't care what your goal is. It could be a goal to just lose five pounds. It could be to get through just one yoga class with taking only four child's poses (the white flag pose of yoga) when you need to instead of taking ten. It could be to play more with your kids, or to be able to pick them up again with little or no strain. It could be able to sit behind your desk to do your job and at the end of the day, to not be on the floor trying to get your back to let go. It could be to drink more water. Eat a piece of fruit or a veggie. I don't care. What matters is that you start doing something. If it helps, write it down. Put friendly reminders in your phone. Say these goals out loud. Think these goals. And when you accomplish these goals, make a note of it. Pause for a brief moment and tell yourself "good job." Show yourself some kindness.

What matters to you? Think about it. You know what your goal is, and you're the only one that needs to know what it is. Now. What are you going to do about it? If you were already doing something that was working for you, you wouldn't be reading this book. *What is the definition of insanity? Doing the same thing over and over again and expecting a different outcome.*

The Don'ts of Yoga

DON'T #1: Don't over think it.

Listen to your gut, your intuition. If it feels "not quite right" then it probably isn't right for you. Take a step back, let off the gas, shift gears and breathe. Pay attention to what your body is telling you. Your body is an extremely smart and amazing machine. If we listen to it and then **DO** as it's requesting (Do #3), we will not have to listen to it later on in the day when it's screaming at us because we chose to ignore it earlier in the day. For me that is one of the hardest things for me to do which is to be okay with my body telling me that I need to take it easy for the day.

DON'T #2: Don't let your ego take over.

Keeping up with the Jones's mentality (I mentioned this earlier) or blaming it on testosterone is lame. Come up with a better story like, "Aliens abducted me last night and planted a chip in my brain that controls my actions. I just had to go into that toe hold stand because they forced me." That sounds a lot more entertaining than, "Even though the instructor said to start at the first modification, I figured I was young and what the hell ... if she can do it, so can I." Which leads me to DON'T #3.

DON'T #3: Don't push yourself too far before you are ready!

Modify your movements! In addition to the rules that I previously gave you, and in the DO #3 of listening to your body, when your body and mind are telling you that you probably should modify, DO it. There are so many who do not have physical issues when they first start yoga, however, after practicing for years, they end up having shoulder issues, or lower back issues. Many times because they think they are stronger than they are and do not modify. *Chatarungas* (basically a plank low to the ground with your elbows in nice and tight) are one of the biggest contributing factors to rotator cuff /shoulder issues. People allow their egos to take over, and instead of keeping their elbows in nice and tight they chicken wing it. Lots of birds in yoga, but chicken is NOT one of them.

DON'T #4: Don't stop moving!

As I just mentioned in DON'T #3 about not pushing yourself too far and that you should modify, some may take that as a cue to stop moving. That is NOT what I said. You need to keep moving. If you need to, take three breaths and then move an appendage. Or shorten your stride. Modify the pose, put your knees on the ground, don't raise your arms so high, or change the angle you are moving them.

Think of it this way. Have you ever seen an injured deer? Do they lay on the side of the road waiting for the EMTs or do they get up and move if they are able? Even if they barely apply any pressure to the leg, or hoof, they keep moving. Why? If they don't, they will be another animal's dinner. It's the same concept for you. You may not be an animal's dinner, but you will be slowly dying. Haven't you heard? Sitting is the new smoking.

DON'T #5: Don't stop doing what is working for you!

I get it. Life is busy and can get in the way. But if you start a yoga practice on a regular basis and you start to feel better, you start to make progress, many times you'll start to let your yoga practice go. It may be because your life is still busy, but many times people stop practicing yoga or other physical activity they were participating in because *they were feeling better*! If you stop practicing yoga or exercising or eating right you stop doing what is working for you to keep you in control of your chronic pain. You stop being proactive. That is one of the biggest mistakes that you can make. So, don't stop doing what is working for you.

DON'T #6: Don't get too caught up in the proper *pranayama* breathing.

Many instructors and meditation practitioners believe that there are better breaths than others and the breath work and mediation is the most important. While that may be true, your goal should be to just keep breathing.

In the beginning when you are first starting to learn yoga, many individuals become overwhelmed. "You want me to put my body in that position and I'm just getting the hang of child's pose?"

If you get too focused on the breath and not the pose you might end up agitating and flaring up your injury or issue. I understand that your goal is to learn to connect the breath to the movement, but in the beginning just try to get the modifications and just keep breathing.

Don't hold your breath and pass out. That would be embarrassing. And it makes me have to do more paperwork.

DON'T #7: Don't rely on others for your success.

Why do I say this? If you tell yourself that you are going to a yoga class because your friend is your yoga buddy, or if you think you'll do yoga once the kids go to bed, then what happens? Your friend bails on you. What a great excuse to skip class! You didn't feel like it anyway. Or your kids stay up longer than usual finishing homework. Whoops! No time for that yoga DVD tonight.

When reaching your goals is contingent on something else happening, or on someone else, no matter good it sounds and how good everyone's intentions are, these turn into excuses that will hinder you obtaining your goal. When you rely on others to hold you accountable, you're setting yourself up for failure. The only one you are ever in control of, is yourself.

You may not be able to control outside resistance called LIFE, but you are in control of how you respond and react to the situation.

It is not anyone else's responsibility to be in charge or to own your pain. When clients and patients would tell me that they didn't do their sun salutations, or their pigeon, even though they have told me that it helps them with their pain, I ask them why not. The typical response I get is that they ran out of time or they were too tired.

Time for more Sam logic:

1. If they are standing there telling me that their pain is so bad, my thought is that they are bullshitting me. Why? I don't know about you, but if I get a headache, migraine or a pain that is so unbearable, you had better believe your ass that I will be doing everything that I can to keep it under control and get rid of it.

2. Bullshit on the time thing. Everyone has time. You're just choosing to spend your time doing other things. If you have five minutes in your day doing anything like sitting behind the steering wheel of your car, sitting at your desk, or at your kid's soccer practice, then you've got time. You can do easy seated spinal twists at your desk, in your car, and you can find a corner of the gym where you could do some sun salutations. It's the ego that is not allowing you to find a corner because you care what others will think of you. Remember, they do not own your pain. Your pain really has no outcome on their lives. So who gives a shit what they think of you doing a little bit of yoga?

So, if you are making that choice to not do what is helping you (Don't #5), then I am thinking you enjoy the attention that you get from complaining about it. Oh, and by the way, if you are, I bet the people that you are always complaining to are tired and fed up with hearing you bitch and moan about it all the time. Or maybe the pain is not really that bad to begin with!?

Let's say that someone else really is the cause of your pain. That you were in an accident, the doctor did screw up, or you were just in the wrong place at the wrong time. It cannot be changed. So now what? You are still in the position/situation you are right now. You can keep living in the past and give in to the thought that the rest of our life has been written for you and it doesn't look good. *Or*, you can take responsibility for your pain and stop blaming others, the medications, the doctors, your family and friends. When you take ownership of your pain and your actions is when you will be able to control your pain. You are in control of your journey in this life.

Go to
www.YogaforChronicPainResources.com
to download a printable pdf of the Dos and Don'ts of Yoga that you can keep on your fridge, next to your TV, or in your car or gym bag for quick reference.

Ownership of Your Actions is Power

I used to think that it didn't matter what I did, that my "path" in this life was already written. I was wrong. I found that out when I decided that I did not like where the road was taking me. I picked up the pen and said, "Screw that. I'm rewriting this shit." Writing and deciding how your future will go is power.

Excuses will not get your chronic pain under control.

However, how may mighty kings fell due to power? Power is a double-edged sword. You now know you are charge and have the power, but if you make the choice to sit your ass on the couch, then you have no one to blame but yourself for your pain later on. That is a scary feeling to know that you will have no one else to blame but yourself. It sucks being an adult sometimes. But guess what? You are not entitled to a pain-free life. That doesn't exist for any of us. If you are alive you will feel pain—mental, emotional and physical.

Having a thought process like this is going to help you to get over that fear of kinesiophobia and your other fears. Yes it will take time and yes, it is a process, but you can do it. You just need to change your perspective. You can do yoga. You just need to find out how to practice what is right for you.

I know that this might seem harsh, but excuses will not get your chronic pain under control. And my thought is that if you are not willing to put some effort and work into getting your body healthier and stronger, then you really are not in that much pain. Because if you were you would be doing everything that you can do get it under control. Is it hard to restart that cycle of movement and function and force yourself up off the couch and to move? Yup. But once again, it's a choice. And you have to make the choice to do it. Every choice has a consequence. Positive or negative, but it has a consequence.

And now that you have made the choice of doing yoga and taking control of your pain, you might find yourself saying, "Holy crap! This yoga thing hurts!" Remember, many times you are just uncomfortable. It's not necessarily pain.

The Great Balancing Act

As I said in the very first chapter, it's all about perspective. If there is a day where you have a flare up or have super low energy, remember one of the best things that you can do for yourself is to *move*. I'm not asking you to do a fast-paced, vinyasa-style practice. I am making the suggestion to go for a walk, get down on the floor, do a pigeon pose, or a couple of cat/cows and "stretch." It's all about perspective.

What do I mean by that? Our society in America tries to sell you the quick fix. The simple, easy not-a-lot-of-effort way of fixing your problem. Don't forget that popping that pill may have about 20 potential worse serious side effects (don't worry your pretty little head about that) but here is an easy way for you to lose weight. Eight-minute abs, a gluten free diet and the list goes on. Look, if you do not have Celiac disease, then why are you going on a gluten free diet? Because it's all the rage in Hollywood? Look at the label on the packages of those products. There are more calories in the gluten free than the real things.

Think of it this way: everything in moderation. If you read and believe in the Bible, it says this. I think it's called gluttony? If you go to extremes many times this will lead to you become out of balance. Vegans seem to have many health problems that they did not have before they went on this very restricted diet. A glass of red wine a day is supposed to be heart healthy, a whole bottle a day ... not a good idea. Everything in moderation. Even exercise can become a compulsive habit for some. Anything can become an obsession, a compulsion if you let it, even yoga.

Life is about balance. Yoga is about balance. The yin and the yang. Physical, mental, emotional and spiritual balance. And when you become out of balance, and you do not listen to your body, it will force you to listen. Whether it manifests itself in weird dreams, or lack of sleep, or other bodily pain, your body will force you to pay attention to it.

And if you practice yoga to the extent you are able to do in this moment, on this day, and then do as your body is requesting, your life will start to become more balanced.

You are an awesome work in progress.

How long with this take? I can't tell you that. Everyone is different. I can tell you that is will more than likely not be as quick as you'd like it. Things happen when you are ready for them by acknowledging them and no longer avoiding them. When you acknowledge what you are trying to run from, that is when you are able to decide what action you will take to address it. Physically, mentally and emotionally. If you force yourself into a something that you are not ready for, physically—let's say a crow (*bakasana*)—then your body will let you know. If you force yourself into something emotionally you are not ready for—let's say a relationship— more than likely your heart will let you know if it will work or not.

It is called a yoga practice because not matter how long we have been practicing yoga we can always benefit and grow from doing it. Yoga is a practice, a tool that you can modify and change to compliment you as you continue on your journey finding your authentic self. It's a process.

Just remember that you are an awesome work in progress, and as long as you keep coming back to your mat, even if it is for ten minutes a day, that is ten minutes longer than not doing it all.

It takes a lot of effort to ignore the body and not listen to it when it is screaming at you to come out of a pose or you're trying to convince yourself to get into a pose. But taking the action in attempting yoga it is the first step in changing your perspective about your chronic pain. Maybe even controlling your chronic pain. What you learn about yourself, how you teach yourself mindfulness in being aware of what is going on with you daily, can help you learn what needs to be addressed and worked on in all areas of your life so you are able to expose and allow your authentic self to emerge and enjoy the adventure.

When you are able to allow your authentic self to emerge with confidence, you can face what is coming your way for that day, that week, and that you can handle life ... your possibilities are endless! You can live the kick ass life you desire and deserve.

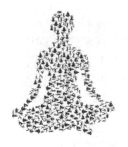

I can accept failure.
Everyone fails at something.
But I cannot accept not trying.
–Michael Jordan

***

Can't is a choice.
–Sam

11

Now Go Forth and Kick Ass!

As you read this book you may have been thinking to yourself that this sounded more like a self-help book more than a book about yoga and chronic pain. I guess you could look at it that way. But you do need to help yourself. Taking ownership of your pain, and how your actions and behaviors play a key role in managing your chronic pain, it's all you. You are helping yourself.

When you take away relying on others and depending on yourself for your happiness and health, this is many times the shift you need to getting back on the path to healing. I am not saying stop taking your doctor's advice and flush your pills down the toilet. I am suggesting that your food choices, exercise habits, sleep routine, yoga practice and your thoughts all play a role in your chronic pain. If you want to start taking over-the-counter supplements or change your diet, ask your medical provider or a nutritionist. Not every supplement is created equal and not every calorie is created equal as well. Get informed. Gain knowledge. Gain power.

When you strip away the layers of chronic pain, you'll often find the root cause keeping you from moving forward. And you may not like what the root cause is. Chronic pain is a complicated thing. It may take multiple different yoga styles, techniques and philosophy concepts to find the best practice for you at this juncture in your life. Living in constant pain can be extremely stressful. Stress can contribute to intensifying your pain daily just by having to deal with your pain. Everyone knows that stress is not good for anyone in general. It can wreak havoc on us.

Perfect example: presidents. I think all of us have seen how quickly a president ages right in front of our eyes. Many times they have little grey and a few wrinkles when they enter office. By the end of the presidency (and especially by the end of back to back terms) they look almost ten or 12 years older. They have heads full of grey hair and a hell of a lot more wrinkles. If you want visible proof that stress has a negative impact on our bodies, just look at pictures of past presidents.

Now think of older popular actresses, models and actors— those that have lived overall healthier active, more nutritious lives—look much younger than they are. Due to yoga, proper nutrition, exercise, sleep, positive thoughts, and more than likely not having to deal with similar stress as you have, these are all factors that help limit the amount of cellular damage on their bodies.

Now before you start jumping my shit again and say these celebrities have it made and I shouldn't be comparing their lives to yours, I will say, yes. They do seem to have it easier. They have cooks, personal trainers, money to spend at the spas and for daily life expenses. They more than likely are not living paycheck to paycheck like you are. You may be correct.

But even with all the money and time they may seem to have, they are still choosing *conscious* positive choices and behaviors on a daily basis to take the time to eat right, to exercise, and to *make* time to decompress physically, mentally and emotionally. They do not do it for short periods of time. They've made these choices their lifestyle habits.

Making New Choices

You might not have the funds to be dropping on a cook, personal trainer and massage therapist, but you do have options in your choices and behaviors that fit into your budget and into your busy schedule in making healthier decisions to combat your chronic pain.

Obesity is one of the leading causes of diabetes, hypertension and the rise of healthcare costs and financial strain on your wallet. I know, here I go again about the weight thing. But this is important. Why is this important? Like I stated in the previous chapters, you are in control of your choices and behaviors. These are all very preventable diseases that are brought on our poor lifestyle habits that lead to being overweight, financial issues and more than likely are contributing to your chronic pain. If your chronic pain is because of something else, I'm sure changing some of your behaviors and choices to healthier ones would benefit you as well.

We may not be able to stop Father Time, but you are able to turn back the hands of time in the way that you age. You are able make your body healthier and younger on a cellular level by changing your choices and behaviors in how you treat your body. And when you start to make your body healthier, you help to heal the wounded areas on your body causing your pain.

The cells that you are producing today are basically brand new. Think of these new cells as young recruits just out of boot camp. They are strong, lean, mean fighting machines with hearts to help, defend and aid those who cannot. If you continue to support them with ammo, feed, train and nurture these new recruits they will support your body and aid in the fight to heal the existing wounds and pain. As they bring aid to the wounded, the wounded cells start to gain strength as they heal. These healthy strong cells become larger in numbers, taking the new healthy cells and the wounded who have now healed and gained strength continue on their crusade of heal and healing with ease.

Remember how I mentioned in Chapter 6 how the fascia encompasses so much more of your body than we thought? And how it changes as your muscular mass changes. These are all cells that are being replaced with strength. Every seven years, basically every cell in your body is brand new. You have an entirely new body every seven years! That is pretty cool. Not pretty cool. Extremely cool!

How you treat your body's health army on a daily basis directly, making sure they are equipped with the right necessities for them to do their jobs correctly, impacts how those cells behave in your body. If your cells are being treating poorly, i.e. taking away their rations and ammo so they have to do hand-to-hand combat, they are not going to be able to do their job effectively. They may win at first, but the extra effort they are exerting as well as having to take time to heal from some punches will take its toll. They will have to rely on their buddies to help, but once these health soldiers are in hand-to-hand combat they will weaken. And if something major happens like North Korea finally figures out how launch missiles more successfully, i.e. a bad cold, flu or accident happens, your health army will already be at a disadvantage bracing for impact and then helping with the cleanup.

This isn't rocket science (pun intended) or anything you haven't heard before, but I've said it before and I will say it again. Making new healthy choices will not be easy. I am not saying this to discourage you. I am saying this to prepare you for battle. The battle in achieving a healthy body, mind, spirit and soul and achieve a kick ass life with as little pain as possible. (Notice I said as little pain, not pain free.)

So now with all of this being said you may be wondering, "This is all great Sam but how do I achieve this kick ass life?"

I don't have all the answers. You don't have all the answers. Many times when we find the answers they will end up changing as we change and grow. So how do we make these new choices?

I know I threw a lot of information at you, so I'll try to hit a few of the highlights that you should be able to easily do that will make big changes for you in a short amount of time. We human like instant gratification. Some of these will provide that for you as well as being fairly easy to implement.

1. Drinking more water. As I've mentioned numerous times throughout this book, this one simple thing can have a huge impact on your cellular health and your chronic pain. Aim for half your body weight in ounces a day. At the very least, drink a little more and more each day until you're at that target. This amount doesn't include your 1:1 ratio – if you drink 10 oz. coffee, you need to drink 10 oz. of water. (That's on top of and in addition to half you're your body weight in ounces a day!) Friendly reminder why. Your vertebrae are like a kitchen sponge. If you're not giving the body enough water, your organs will suck it from your soft tissues (your muscles and scar tissue), leaving them dehydrated and brittle, and more prone to injury. The human body is roughly 60 percent water. The brain and heart around 70 percent and the lungs about 80 percent all give or take. If you are dehydrated and there is not enough water surrounding the brain just visualize what happens when it starts to shrivel up?! (I'm not saying that is what happens. Just trying to get across the point that water is important!)

2. Getting some exercise. Remember, movement counts. Exercise doesn't have to be lifting weights at the gym. Go outside for a hike or a walk. Do *something*. Park your car farther away from the entrance to work or into the store. Go kick the soccer ball with your kids. If you are not exercising you are limiting the amount of blood flow, oxygen, nutrients to your body the best way possible. It's as simple as that. Your body heals by having these things get to the muscles, the organs, and the other many parts of your body.

If you exercise you are stimulating those cells and creating a more efficient way to help your body heal and keeping you healthy in general. Preventative medicine. When your body is able to receive the things that it needs more quickly it can utilize those resources at a much faster pace which will lead to the cells becoming happier and healthier. The healthier your cells are, the longer you will live. Not to mention, you'll like the way you look and feel, boosting your self-esteem—

then you'll likely want to stay active because the cute guy in your spin class keeps looking your way, and your butt is looking better in your jeans. And you're sleeping better!

3. Get more sleep! I just mentioned it. The average adult needs an average of seven to nine hours of sleep. Sleep helps us to repair cellular damage we have done deliberately or that's caused by the environment. It helps to recharge the body and the brain. Our brain is the body's hard drive. It needs to be able to fire off billions of nerve cells that coordinate our thoughts, movement, behaviors, sensations and emotions to name a few. If it hasn't been able to recharge properly then you cannot expect it to operate your body efficiently throughout the day. I fully get that getting more sleep is looked at as a luxury with all we have to do but try to go to bed just 30 minutes earlier. Read a book. (I highly recommend the one you are reading.) And try to turn off electronics about 30 minutes prior to going to sleep as well. The sound and light do trigger the sensory neurons in the brain and make it think it needs to pay attention when it really needs to be resting.

4. Eating what fuels your body most. I know this one you may have been working on for a while and you do not think it is easy. I agree. So please think about it this way. For those that are car people, if you put diesel fuel in a car that takes unleaded what is going to happen to your engine? It's going to get stuck and not run efficiently. Same concept with your body. Yet we constantly are eating things that are made in a lab that our body is not designed to break down. It does eventually break it down (or at least most of it) because it is forced to. And your body has to work harder to do it. I bet that your body is definitely not running as optimally as it could be. I know it's not. You don't have to go to extremes.

Here is a simple easy step you can take. Have you ever heard, eat breakfast like a king, lunch like a prince, dinner like a pauper? You need fuel throughout your day so your car/body can go. It does not need much fuel when it is parked in the garage or in bed for the night. Oh, and eat your veggies. Even if you increase it to just one more veggie a day that is a good start.

5. Doing yoga (of course!). How about trying yoga? Or trying it again with the info you have learned from this book? Yoga can be one of the first decisions you make in achieving the life you desire and controlling your chronic pain. And it does not have to be a 60 to 90-minute-long class right out the gate. Try finding a free yoga classes in your area or a beginner class. With the information that I supplied you in this book you should be able to implement these key things even while practicing from a YouTube video from your home. (I have been asked numerous times to put up videos, so, ask and you shall receive. It's in the works.)

Yoga helps us to step away from the crazy and decompress from daily stress.

Yoga can help us learn more about ourselves and this self-awareness helps us to implement the different thought patterns, habits and movement that you want to change. These small conscious healthy choices start a positive health cycle. The more you consciously make these new and healthy decisions they start to travel the dirt road and create a rut filled with gold. A new neuropathway that you unconsciously and naturally start travel without thinking about it in making healthier choices. Yoga helps us to step away from the crazy and decompress from daily stress. To shut the world out even if it's for an hour or so. To pay attention to ourselves. To put us at the top of the priority list for an hour. To help us focus on our needs, our wants, and to just be. This a way that we can show ourselves kindness. Discovering your authentic self and showing it kindness is so important and key for those that have chronic pain.

Since you now know that you can change the way that your cells function and that moving is a positive way you can actually lessen your pain, wouldn't you try it? The only thing you have to lose is fat! And possibly chronic pain. You may have muscle soreness, but that is an awesome thing. That muscle soreness is your body's way of letting you know that you have not wasted your time. The good thing about muscle soreness is that in 24 to 72 hours later, it will be gone. When that muscle soreness is gone all it's leaving behind is a healthier happier more efficient functioning body. It's all about perspective.

I personally feel that yoga can help anyone. I have seen yoga be used as a tool to help so many with multiple medical issues. I have seen yoga help athletes who just want to perform better, have seen yoga help athletes keep their careers longer, as well as seeing yoga help an injured athlete reduce their recovery time in half so they can get back more quickly doing what they love.

If what is holding you back from practicing yoga is your fear, I can relate. I stated doing yoga to help with chronic migraines that would lay me out for days. I was young, on medication that I was told I would have to take for the rest of my life and had small kids who did not understand how to make Mommy's boo boo better. I was fearful that this was going to be a constant the rest of my life.

I was then fearful of practicing yoga and then I was fearful when I started teaching that I was not a good yoga instructor. I know I don't fit into the mold of what a yoga instructor should be like. I have felt like odd man out most of my life. Especially as a yoga instructor. I have been told often, "You're not what I pictured when I think of yoga instructors." I curse. I joke. I can be a bit harsh. I should be calmer, especially since I practice yoga. I get that a lot. I tell them just think of what I would be like if I didn't!

I have learned to take these comments as a compliment. (I can spin anything into a positive.) I get that I am not everyone's cup of tea. And that is okay as there are hundreds of other good instructors out there who will be the right teacher for them. I have learned to embrace and to allow my authentic self to emerge and come out of hiding. I have learned that all of the years I was hiding my authentic self I missed out on learning more about who I am while trying to please and be someone who was not going to accept my authentic self. And for what?

Please, I would like you to be open minded to the thought process of trying yoga. There are many good yoga instructors that teach a way and a style that you will be able to relate to. But it may take time to find the right combo of instructor and style. Some love the instructor but hate the style of yoga they teach. Some love the style of yoga but can't stand the instructor's voice or the way they breathe.

If you've been practicing yoga and are still on the hunt for that perfect combo of instructor and style, keep in mind some of the ideas, thoughts and perspectives I introduced to you throughout this book. They will help keep you fairly safe and help you keep moving in your journey. If other styles and forms of yoga weren't or aren't working for you, give this a try. What have you got to lose? When you are open minded to different thoughts, ideas and people, you never know when you might learn. It could be something about your job, your family, friends, or most importantly ... yourself.

Can Yoga Save Your Life?

I have heard many times from yoga instructors and others who practice yoga *"yoga saved my life."* As much as I believe they are coming from a sincere place and truly believe that this individual feels this strongly about how yoga helped them, they are selling themselves short. I personally do not believe that yoga *"saved their lives."* Yoga was a tool that the individual used. The *individual* saved her own life.

The individual took action and made countless, conscious choices to change their behaviors to achieve their desired outcomes. I would bet money that these individuals make other conscious choices about their lifestyle habits—their sleep routine, their nutrition (notice I did not say diet?), their work conditions, their family, friends, and the many other life decisions that impact their lives daily. These all play a role in our overall health, wellbeing and chronic pain.

It was a combination of the individual doing the work, of being honest with themselves and to stop running from their fears. It was the individual making the conscious continuous decision to keep taking the steps of going to a yoga class, and to keep going back. Of making the conscious continuous healthier decisions about their daily habits, behaviors and thoughts. It took effort. It took determination and it took time.

Those that "get saved" did not have it happen overnight. If a particular yoga style did not work for them, they tried a different style, or a different teacher. It was that individual making the mental and conscious choices to help build and create a new healthier, happier life and not giving up on the possibility of a better quality of life for them and their families.

The individual took the time, put forth the effort, the energy and did not give up when their bodies were screaming at them to do so. Instead they moved how they could in that moment on that day.

Yoga is more than breathing, headstands and touching your toes.

Yoga was a catalyst to help them be more mindful of their eating, their sleep, and their water intake. The individual was being proactive, not reactive. They may have even tried different modalities like acupuncture, massage or a chiropractor or (gasp) eating more fruits and veggies or drinking more water!

It does take time and effort in finding our unique and "perfect" cocktail of health. And it's well worth the effort! I can speak first hand and attest to that. Yoga is a tool that has helped so many individuals reach goals that they set for themselves. Yoga was the resource that may have provided a sense of belonging with a group of individuals experiencing similar life events and were like-minded. This sense of belonging may have provided the safe environment to let go of their fears and allow their authentic selves to emerge.

Yoga is more than breathing, headstands and touching your toes. Yoga is about learning about yourself. Your strengths, your weaknesses. Yoga helps us learn about who we really are, what we truly desire physically, mentally, and emotionally. Yoga is about becoming more self-aware and learning to be *honest* with yourself about what and how we are feeling. Yoga helps us to become aware of how we are changing on a daily basis. And when we are aware of the changes that are happening within us, even though life gets crazy and stressful, we have a better understanding of our fears that feed our chronic pain. And with better understanding comes a better understanding of learning how to combat and manage our chronic pain.

Becoming aware and honest about who we truly are, I think is the most difficult and challenging thing to do, but it may actually be the easiest part of the journey. Letting go of the ego is the tricky part, for me at least, and actually doing as the body, mind and heart are requesting. *Not* what society or our yoga classmates, peers and loved ones are doing or telling us what we should be doing, but *what we know in our guts and heart* we should be doing for ourselves.

The actions that we know we should be taking, and then not taking mostly due to fear, is scary. It's unknown territory. What happens if it doesn't work? What happens if you are wrong, and your body really wants you to do this instead of that? Half of figuring out what does work, is figuring out what doesn't work. If you don't take the action, you won't find out.

There is a fine line about wanting to quit. To stop moving and giving up when you have a flare up. Or you have a physical setback. It hard when you're having an emotionally draining day. But this happens to all of us in our lives. Even for those that are not dealing with chronic pain. It's called life.

And when all we want to do is sit our asses on the couch because it's just easier and we are exhausted, this is the most important time that we need to move!

We all need yoga. I don't care who you are, what your sex, age, height, weight, injury, or other medical (mental and physical) issues are, you can do yoga. You have just not been able to have yoga explained to you in a way that fits your needs, or more importantly shown how to do the poses correctly.

The key is to try to find the style, mediation and yoga practice that works best for you. There is no one size fits all. Hell, yoga may not be a fit for you. So, if you want to call it stretching, or dynamic warm ups, I don't care. Just *move*!!

If there was a magic pill, or the perfect workout, or the perfect "diet," whoever created it would be a billionaire 100 times over and we would be living happier and healthier lives with a quick fix.

Quick fixes are temporary. Quick fixes do not last. Quick fixes are marketing gimmicks. Quick fixes are how companies are able to sell you their product. Quick fixes are a fairy tale. They tell you what you want to hear. Not what is real.

If nothing else, I hope that you have gained better insight how to implement the basics and fundamentals to help protect and inform yourself as you start or continue on your yoga journey to help with your chronic pain. Or to be able to take some of these underlying ways of keeping yourself safe and apply them to other physical activities.

I hope that I've at least given you the confidence enough to start asking your medical providers more questions. To learn more about your medical issue. To talk with your peers, friends and family about what is going on with you. To ask questions of your yoga instructors, Pilates instructors and personal trainers and to be more proactive in your overall wellbeing. If you do not really understand what they are telling you, or why you should be doing things the way they say, it is okay to keep asking questions until you do have a better understanding.

You are in control of your life. You can take back control of your chronic pain.

I will say this. We are all human. There are super amazing intelligent people who dedicate their entire lives to learning science and trying to make the work a better place by helping heal and alleviate pain. However, they are human. And sometimes they do not have all of the answers. It is not to say that they will not give you great information and knowledge. But it is okay if your gut just doesn't feel like something is right to get a second opinion. To get a third opinion. And if your provider says you are foolish to do so if that is what you feel is right for you … you might need a new medical provider.

I would love to hear from you about how you're using the tools and techniques from this book in your yoga practice and your life. Please send me an email at sam.parker@neotericmovementsystems.com and be sure to check out the Learn More page at the end of this book to connect with me on social media and find out about workshops and trainings to dive deeper into yoga for chronic pain.

If you walk away from this book with nothing else, I hope that you walk away with an attitude that *you* are in control of your chronic pain.

You are in control of your life. You can take back control of your chronic pain. You can take back control of your life so you are able to achieve the life that you want. It will be hard. It will be challenging. You will have set backs. But you can do it. And it will take time. The question now becomes you *going* to do it?

You have the power. You now have greater knowledge and tools.

Now go forth and kick ass!!

REFERENCES

[1] Treede, R.-D., Rief, W., Barkc, A., Aziz, Q., Bennett, M. I., Benoliel, R., Wang, S.-J. (2015). A classification of chronic pain for *ICD-11*. *Pain,* *156*(6), 1003–1007. http://doi.org/10.1097/j.pain.0000000000000160

[2] Current Concepts in Muscle Stretching For Exercise And Rehabilitation. International Journal of Sports Physical Therapy, 7(1), 109–119.

[3] Knapik, A., Saulicz, E., & Gnat, R. (2011). Kinesiophobia – Introducing a New Diagnostic Tool. Journal of Human Kinetics, 28, 25–31.

[4] Burns, L. C., Ritvo, S. E., Ferguson, M. K., Clarke, H., Seltzer, Z., & Katz, J. (2015). Pain catastrophizing as a risk factor for chronic pain after total knee arthroplasty: a systematic review. Journal of Pain Research, 8, 21–32.

[5] H. Susan J. Picavet, Johan W. S. Vlaeyen, Jan S. A. G. Schouten; Pain Catastrophizing and Kinesiophobia: Predictors of Chronic Low Back Pain , American Journal of Epidemiology, Volume 156, Issue 11, 1 December 2002, Pages 1028–1034.

LEARN MORE

Thank you for taking the time to read this book. I know from personal experience how yoga can change people's lives, and really give them back the life they thought they'd lost due to chronic pain. My goal was to give you insights into why you might still be in pain long after an injury has healed, and give you some strategies to help you incorporate yoga into your pain management plan. Honestly, if I've been able to help you make one positive shift in your yoga practice, or helped you diminish your chronic pain, I would love to hear about it at sam.parker@neotericmovementsystems.com.

I believe in you! You are the sole reason I wrote this book. I'm passionate about helping you combat your chronic pain and create the happy, healthy life you deserve. I want to support you in any way I can. I've been blessed to connect with incredible coaches and teachers as I've grown as a yogi and I'm serious about paying it forward!

I invite you to use the touch-points below to stay connected. Use them to celebrate your triumphs, learn from your failures, and to voice your frustrations or challenges from a place of openness and curiosity, so that others facing similar obstacles realize they aren't alone.

Staying Connected

Instagram: @samanthaparker_nms

Facebook: @NeotericMovementSystems

Email: sam.parker@neotericmovementsystems.com

Online Resources

Sign up at www.YogaforChronicPainResources.com for access to downloads and get updates on new programs and events.

If you're a yoga instructor, find out about Sam's training programs and CME courses at:
www.neotericmovementsystems.co/pages/continued-medical-education-cmes/

Finding a Certified Yoga Therapist

If you'd like to seek out a yoga instructor with more knowledge, look for someone with the C-IAYT designation, which means they're a certified yoga therapist. These yoga therapists have a much deeper understanding of anatomy and physiology, more in-depth training in yoga, and many times have healthcare licenses. Please go to www.iayt.com to find a certified yoga therapist near you.

ABOUT THE AUTHOR

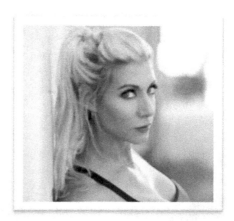

Samantha Parker is a certified yoga therapist (C-IAYT) with a B.S. in Sports and Exercise Science, currently pursuing her master's degree in kinesiology. A certified personal trainer, she has taught over 5,000 hours of yoga on three different continents, helping thousands of patients.

For four years, Samantha was the Chief Movement Therapist at Landstuhl Regional Medical Center—the largest military hospital outside the U.S.—in the Interdisciplinary Pain Management Center.

There she created, implemented and performed research for the first yoga program in a new U.S. Army initiative for chronic pain rehabilitation.

Samantha is also a founding member of the Special Operations Fortitude Center (SOF-C), which helps various U.S. Special Operations Forces troops recover from mild traumatic brain injuries, chronic pain and PTSD. In addition to working with military special ops forces, she has also worked with professional athletes from football players to ballet dancers.